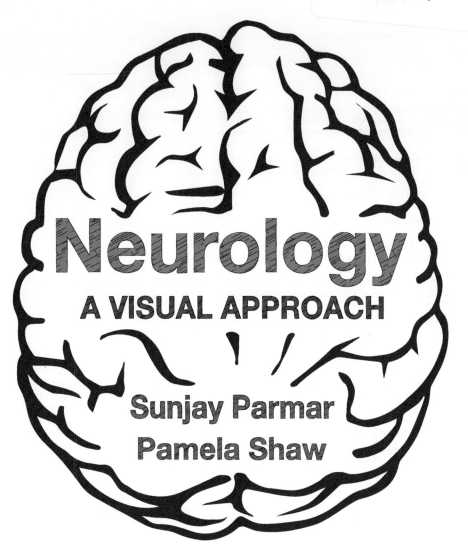

Neurology
A VISUAL APPROACH

Sunjay Parmar
Pamela Shaw

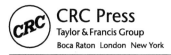

CRC Press
Taylor & Francis Group
Boca Raton London New York

CRC Press is an imprint of the
Taylor & Francis Group, an **informa** business

CRC Press
Taylor & Francis Group
6000 Broken Sound Parkway NW, Suite 300
Boca Raton, FL 33487-2742

Printed on acid-free paper

International Standard Book Number-13: 978-1-138-04376-3 (Hardback)
International Standard Book Number-13: 978-1-4987-8206-7 (Paperback)

Visit the Taylor & Francis Web site at
http://www.taylorandfrancis.com

and the CRC Press Web site at
http://www.crcpress.com

CONTENTS

FOREWORD

Neurology is often viewed by medical students as a difficult subject to learn. Due to the complexity of the nervous system, learning about all the different neurological disorders and their clinical features and management can seem daunting at first. However, neurology is one of the most fascinating subjects and it is important for all doctors to master the basic elements of this subject, given that around 20% of medical emergencies are neurological. In this book we have approached the subject in an unorthodox manner, using visual imagery to portray the key features of common neurological conditions to stimulate interest, learning and further investigation. Multiple research studies have shown that this approach facilitates enhanced recall and long-term retention of subject matter. The material in this book is up-to-date with current guidelines, making this an accessible resource that readers will want to pick up again and again, whilst having fun in the process.

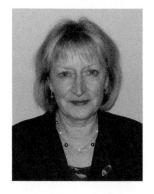

This is a one-of-a-kind text, and I look forward to further works from this imaginative and talented young doctor. We hope that the contents of this book will represent a welcome surprise, especially to readers looking for smarter ways to absorb important information quickly.

Professor Dame Pamela Shaw

PREFACE

Neurology: A visual approach is a study book designed to help readers quickly learn and remember pertinent, high-yield information about a comprehensive range of neurological conditions through pictorial representation.

Much of our memory is created from images. Drawing from my experience in participating in memory competitions and being an honorary teacher in medical education, this book has been specifically designed to increase the rate of knowledge acquisition as well as long-term retention, whilst making the process of learning fun through the use of humour and exaggeration (both well-known and effective memory adjuncts). This places the book ideally as a quick revision resource for upcoming examinations and learning in the ward environment. The pages are arranged in an easy to follow layout, with the visual mnemonic (representation of a condition with all key facts encoded into pictures) and associated legend on the left, and a high-yield one-page review of each condition (covering definition and aetiology to management and prognosis) on the right.

Visual mnemonics are a great way to assimilate and recall information quickly. However, first and foremost, knowledge should be learned conceptually, knowing the real nuts and bolts of something rather than superficial learning. This small text is not meant to be a total solution for your revision needs but rather an effective adjunct to help provide an efficient and more stimulating method of learning.

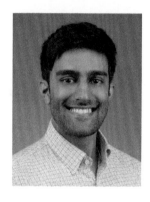

An end goal of this book is to change your perception of what learning means to you. Ideally, this text will act as a gateway that will help you to create your own visual mnemonics that you can learn from and share with others. I wish you all the best in your studying endeavours.

Dr Sunjay Parmar

ACKNOWLEDGEMENTS

I am indebted to all those who made this book possible.

I would like to express my upmost gratitude to Professor Pamela Shaw, who saw the potential in this ambitious project, and provided invaluable amendments and insight into the many iterations of the manuscript. Furthermore, my sincere thanks to Dr Saadnah Naidu (my lovely wife), Riddhi Prajapati and Mukund Prajapati for their time in proofreading the manuscript and constructive feedback.

I am grateful for all the support of my colleagues at Taylor & Francis, in particular Dr Joanna Koster, for her support through the initial stages of the book proposal and Kate Nardoni for her help in preparing the manuscript. Finally, I dedicate this book to my parents, without whom I would not be the man I am today. Sai Ram.

I would appreciate any corrections, clarifications or suggestions for future editions. You can contact me at: sunjayparmar@doctors.org.uk

HOW TO USE THIS BOOK

This book has taken the phrase 'a picture is worth a thousand words' literally. If you are new to learning in a visual format, it can be daunting at first glance to know where to start. Below is a guide to help you, whether you are a beginner or a seasoned visual learner.

Teaching by example is the best way to start learning a skill. We will use the visual mnemonic below for Guillain–Barré syndrome, and walk through how to learn the picture step by step. I have gone into a lot of detail to outline the steps; however, very quickly the process of remembering a new visual mnemonic robustly should not take more than 20–30 seconds.

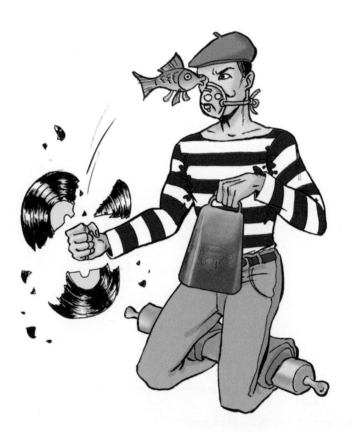

A Frenchman is wearing a green beret	**Guillain–Barré syndrome** Green beret = Guillain–Barré
He is holding cowbell in his left hand	***Campylobacter jejuni*** 'Cowbell' sounded out loosely sounds like *Campylobacter*
A fish is attached to his right eye	**Miller Fisher syndrome**
His legs are wound around a rolling pin and moving up	**Symmetrical ascending lower limb weakness**
He has profuse sweating under his armpits	**Autonomic dysfunction**
He is wearing an oxygen mask	**Respiratory compromise**
A vinyl album disc is being crushed with his right hand	**Albuminocytological dissociation** Album = albuminocytological; disc = dissociation

❶ Briefly scan the picture and sequentially note the association as shown by the picture legend.

- The most important association is the name of the condition with the picture, so whenever you encounter the condition, the picture of the Frenchman in the green beret should automatically come to the forefront of your mind.

❷ Look at each association in turn as shown in the picture legend, and make sure you are certain that it makes sense and is memorable to you; that if you were to look at the picture association, you could remember the corresponding fact.

- If you find that the link is not memorable, feel free to create your own. The beauty of this method is that is it personal to you, so using anything that will encourage a better link is strongly advised.

❸ Learn the picture by building it up one association at a time, instead of learning the picture as a whole.
  - **When imagining, think BIG, exaggerate (movements, colours, emotions) and utilise as many senses (sight, hearing, smell, taste, touch) as possible. These alone are essential to developing a strong visual memory.**

- Image a blank canvas with the man and nothing else linked to him (no fish, no rolling pin, etc.). You can have your eyes open or closed; your preference.

- Add him holding a cowbell: think how shiny it would look; glaring perhaps? Imagine the loud ringing of the cowbell. How does the cowbell feel – cold to the touch? Does it smell of cow manure? Is it being swung rapidly or slowly? Take a moment to fix these different aspects to the Frenchman holding the cowbell. Once you can clearly remember that the man is holding the cowbell in his left hand, move on.

- Add the rolling pin: imagine the excruciating pain he must be in with his legs wound around it. Think about the sounds it would have made being rolled up, possibly the crunching of bones? Does the rolling pin have splinters that are digging into his legs? Does it smell of flour? Exaggerate and use as many senses as possible.

- Add the sweating armpits: imagine how he must be feeling, unable to move because of the wound-up rolling pin and the sticky sensation of his profuse sweating. Imagine the smell – not a nice thought, but now it will be difficult to forget his sweaty armpits. Use anything to increase the memory potential of the links.

- Repeat the process for all remaining associations. After every two links you add, refresh your memory on what links have already been added; so after the sweaty armpits, recall that he is holding a cowbell and his legs are wound around a rolling pin.

❹ Now you have the complete picture memorised. Next, you are going to solidify it in your long-term memory. This is done by recalling the information in different ways. You don't have to do them all, but the additive effect of recalling in multiple ways will really improve the speed of recall and the long-term strength of the association.

- Speak out loud: imagine the picture. Then scan each section of his body from top to bottom. So, first his face. You should be able to remember the fish on his right eye; say out loud 'Miller Fisher syndrome'. Next is the oxygen mask; say out loud 'Respiratory compromise'. Continue downwards, and so on.

- Draw it from memory: get a blank piece of paper. I use an A4 whiteboard; probably the best investment I have ever made. Draw out the picture (stick men are fine), but it is important in your mind to remember the vivid colours, exaggerated features and the sensual information to further consolidate it.

- Create a short story: warning; it can be great fun! The aim is to create a story that can tie in all the links the Frenchman has on him, so going through the story enables you to remember all the links. More imaginative → more memorable.

❺ Spaced repetition: space out your learning. Revisiting revision material at increasing time intervals rather than in large chunks leads to a stronger long-term memory and, interestingly, less total time spent revising.

- There are many approaches to implementing spaced repetition learning, such as using computer software or physical flashcards. With this book, I would recommend a variation of the Leitner system. In this you use any recall method(s) described above to remember the picture, then 1 day after recall again. If successful, recall in 3 days, then 1 week, 2 weeks, 1 month, 3 months. Each time the interval increases.

- If you find a particular visual mnemonic difficult to remember, for example on the 1 week recall, go back to the start and strengthen the association using the above techniques. Then recall again after 3 days, 1 week and so on. Doing this, you will spend less time on things you remember easily and more time on things you don't, which is the way learning should be.

Do not feel dejected if, on first attempts, you forget one or a few parts of the picture. Any skill worth learning does not always start off easy. Learning faster and smarter with visual mnemonics is an attainable skill.

Having personally spoken with many Grandmasters of memory and World Memory Champions, I learned that even they had rocky starts before the automatic nature of the techniques they learnt (which are primarily visual mnemonics) made it faster and easier to retain information.

ABBREVIATIONS

+ve positive

−ve negative

1° primary

2° secondary

3,4-DAP 3,4-diaminopyridine

5-HT$_2$ 5-hydroxytryptamine 2 receptor

Ab antibody

ACA anterior cerebral artery

ACh acetylcholine

AChE acetylcholinesterase

AD Alzheimer's disease

ADEM acute disseminated encephalomyelitis

ADPKD autosomal dominant polycystic kidney disease

AED antiepileptic drug

AF atrial fibrillation

AFB acid-fast bacilli

AFP α-fetoprotein

AICA anterior inferior cerebellar artery

AIDP acute inflammatory demyelinating polyneuropathy

aka also known as

ALS amyotrophic lateral sclerosis

AMAN acute motor axonal neuropathy

AMSAN acute motor–sensory axonal neuropathy

ANA antinuclear antibodies

ApoE4 apolipoprotein E4

APP amyloid precursor protein

ARAS Ascending reticular activating system

ASA anterior spinal artery

ATM ataxia telangiectasia mutated gene

ATP adenosine triphosphate

AV atrioventricular

BBB blood–brain barrier

BD twice daily

BiPAP bilevel positive airway pressure

BP blood pressure

C/I contraindicated

Ca^{2+} calcium

C–C fistula carotid–cavernous fistula

CCB calcium channel blocker

CGRP calcitonin gene-related peptide

CH cluster headache

chr. chromosome

CJD Creutzfeldt–Jakob disease

CK creatine kinase

CMT Charcot–Marie–Tooth disease

CMV cytomegalovirus

CN cranial nerve

CNS central nervous system

CO carbon monoxide

CoA coenzyme A

COCP combined oral contraceptive pill

COMT catechol-O-methyl transferase

CSF cerebrospinal fluid

CT computed tomography

CXR chest X-ray

DAP diaminopyridine

DaTSCAN ioflupane iodine-123 injection

DBS deep brain stimulation

DIC disseminated intravascular coagulation

DMPK dystrophia myotonia protein kinase

DNA deoxyribonucleic acid

DTR deep tendon reflexes

DVLA Driver and Vehicle Licensing Agency (UK)

E. coli Escherichia coli

EBV Epstein–Barr virus

ECG electrocardiogram

Echo echocardiogram

EEG electroencephalogram

EMG electromyography

ESR erythrocyte sedimentation rate

FBC full blood count

FDG-PET fluorodeoxyglucose-positron emission tomography

FLAIR fluid-attenuated inversion recovery (MRI)

FTD frontotemporal dementia

FVC forced vital capacity

GABA γ-aminobuytric acid

GBS Guillain–Barré syndrome

GCS Glasgow coma scale

GI gastrointestinal

GNAQ guanine nucleotide-binding protein G(q) subunit alpha

GTP guanosine triphosphate

h hour

Hb haemoglobin

HBV hepatitis B virus

HCM hypertrophic cardiomyopathy

HD Huntington's disease

HIF1a hypoxia inducible factor 1a

HIV human immunodeficiency virus

HLA human leukocyte antigen

HR heart rate

HSV herpes simplex virus

HTN hypertension

HZV herpes zoster virus

ICA internal carotid artery

ICP intracranial pressure

ID infectious diseases

Ig immunoglobulin

IIH idiopathic intracranial hypertension

IM intramuscular

IOP intra-ocular pressure

IQ intelligence quotient

ITU intensive treatment unit

IV intravenous

IVIG intravenous immunoglobulin

K⁺ potassium

LA local anaesthetic

LAM pulmonary lymphangioleiomyomatosis

L-DOPA L-3,4-dihydroxyphenylalanine

LEMS Lambert–Eaton myasthenic syndrome

LFT liver function tests

LMN lower motor neuron

LMWH low-molecular weight heparin

LOC loss of consciousness

LP lumbar puncture

m/o months old

MAO monoamine oxidase

MC&S microscopy, culture and sensitivity

MCA middle cerebral artery

MCV mean cell volume

MDT multi-disciplinary team

Mg²⁺ magnesium

MI myocardial infarction

min minute

MMA middle meningeal artery

MMSE mini-mental state examination

MND motor neuron disease

MPTP 1-methyl-4-phenyl-1,2,3,6-tetrahydropyridine

MRI magnetic resonance imaging

MS multiple sclerosis

MTB *Mycobacterium tuberculosis*

MuSK muscle specific kinase

N&V nausea and vomiting

N. meningitidis Neisseria meningitidis (meningococcus)

N₂O nitrous oxide

NA noradrenaline

Na⁺ sodium

NF1 neurofibromatosis Type 1

NF2 neurofibromatosis Type 2

NIHSS NIH stroke scale

NMDA N-methyl-D-aspartate

NMJ neuromuscular junction

NSAID non-steroidal anti-inflammatory drug

nvCJD new variant Creutzfeldt–Jakob disease

O$_2$ oxygen

OD once daily

ODS osmotic demyelination syndrome

OT occupational therapist

PCA posterior cerebral artery

PCR polymerase chain reaction

PD Parkinson's disease

PDH pyruvate dehydrogenase

PEG percutaneous endoscopic gastrostomy

PHN post-herpetic neuralgia

PICA posterior inferior cerebellar artery

PMP-22 peripheral myelin protein 22

PPA primary progressive aphasia

PrP prion protein

PSP progressive bulbar palsy

PT physiotherapist

QDS four times daily

RAPD relative afferent pupillary defect

RBC red blood cells

RCC renal cell carcinoma

RCT randomised controlled trials

REZ root entry zone

RTA road-traffic accident

S. pneumoniae Streptococcus pneumoniae (pneumococcus)

s second

SAH subarachnoid haemorrhage

SALT speech and language therapist

SDH subdural haemorrhage/haematoma

SEGA subependymal giant cell astrocytoma

SIADH syndrome of inappropriate antidiuretic hormone secretion

SOB shortness of breath

SOD superoxide dismutase

SSRI selective serotonin reuptake inhibitor

SUDEP sudden death in epilepsy

T1DM type 1 diabetes mellitus

TB tuberculosis

TCA tricyclic antidepressant

TDS three times a day

TFT thyroid function tests

TN trigeminal neuralgia

tPA tissue plasminogen activator

U&E urea and electrolytes

UMN upper motor neuron

USS ultrasound

UV ultraviolet

VGCC voltage-gated calcium channels

VGKC voltage-gated potassium channels

VHL von Hippel–Lindau

VNS vagus nerve stimulation

VP ventriculo-peritoneal

VZV varicella zoster virus

WBC white blood cells

WCC white cell count

WFNS World Federation of Neurological Surgeons

wk week

y/o years old

ZNF9 zinc finger protein 9

ALZHEIMER'S DISEASE

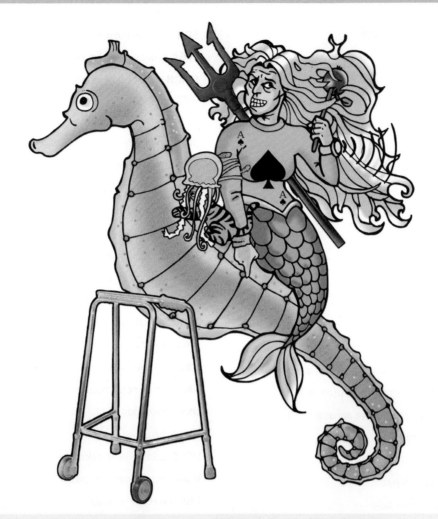

An old lady is on a seahorse with a Zimmer frame, carrying a demon trident	**Alzheimer's disease, old age, dementia** Al'zheimer' = 'Zimmer' frame; old age; demon = dementia
Her hair is very tangled	**Neurofibrillary tangles**
She is holding a toffee apple tangled in her hair	**APP** Apple = APP
She is showing teeth with yellow plaques	**β-amyloid plaques**
She is wearing a jumper decorated with the Ace of spades	**ACh depletion** Ace = ACh
She is riding a seahorse	**Hippocampus** Hippocampus = Greek for seahorse
An ethernet cable is wrapped around her right arm	**ApoE4 variant** Ethernet sounds similar to 'E-four'-net
She is pointing down with her right hand	**Down's syndrome**
She is trying to comb her hair with the apple, not realising the apple is not a comb	**Apraxia, agnosia**
A cat has a stinging jellyfish on its head	**CT, rivastigmine** Cat = CT scan, sting-ing jellyfish = riva-stig-mine
The lady is wearing a vibration alarm watch	**Alarm** (memory aids)
She has a mermaid's lower body	**Memantine**

ALZHEIMER'S DISEASE

DEFINITION
A progressive neurodegenerative disease with global decline in cognition without impairment of consciousness

AETIOLOGY
The majority are sporadic
- Pathophysiology:
  - Tau protein (maintains neuronal cytoskeleton) is normally phosphorylated. Tau protein mutation → hyperphosphorylation → tau proteins become unstable and clump together = **neurofibrillary tangles** → damage neuronal structural integrity. Tangles correlate with dementia severity
  - **APP** is a transmembrane protein (with a role in neuron regulation). Mutation → abnormal APP cleavage → forms β-amyloid; combines into **β-amyloid plaques** → lead to neuronal death; especially cholinergic fibres (hence why ↓ACh). Starts in the **hippocampus**, then progresses to the cortex
- Risk factors:
  - **Age** (largest risk factor), prior intellectual level
  - Genetics:
    - Early onset; autosomal dominant; point mutations in genes associated with amyloid processing: *APP*, *PS1* on chr. 14 and *PS2* on chr. 1)
    - Late-onset (non-familial); **ApoE4 variant**
  - **Down's syndrome** (*APP* on chr. 21; Down's = trisomy 21; 3 copies of *APP* → ↑β-amyloid plaque formation)

EPIDEMIOLOGY
- Most common cause of **dementia** (60–80% of all dementias)
- Affects 5% of >65 y/o. Incidence ↑**exponentially with age**

PRESENTATION
- '5 As' presenting in a steady decline. If they occur abruptly, consider vascular dementia:
  - Anterograde amnesia: forgetfulness is usually the first presenting sign
  - **Agnosia**: inability to recognise/identify objects despite intact sensory function
  - **Apraxia**: impaired ability to carry out motor activities despite intact muscle strength
  - Abnormal executive functioning: impaired planning, organising, abstracting

- Aphasia: language disturbance, typically spared until later

INVESTIGATIONS
- A diagnosis of exclusion; definitively diagnosed only on autopsy
- Bloods: dementia screen; B_{12}, U&E, thyroid function, syphilis serology (if appropriate)
- **CT**/MRI: may see gross anatomical changes, excludes treatable space-occupying lesions:
  - Diffuse cortical atrophy, leading to widened sulci and narrowed gyri
  - Hydrocephalus ex vacuo: ventricles enlarge due to brain atrophy, not due to ↑CSF
- Use MMSE and Wechsler adult IQ scale to help assess severity:
  - MMSE: <27 qualifies for dementia; however, premorbid intellectual function needs to be taken into account
- Psychometric testing: distinguishes dementia from depression (depressive pseudo-dementia)

MANAGEMENT
- Largely supportive:
  - MDT approach is paramount; supportive therapy for patients and family
  - Treatment of associated symptoms: depression, agitation and sleep disturbances
  - Adaptations: memory aids (diaries, labels), **alarms**
    - Prevent disease progression; start medication if MMSE >12 (if <12, the drug side-effects outweigh the benefits):
  - 1st line/mild-moderate: AChE inhibitors, e.g. **rivastigmine**; ↑ACh levels
  - 2nd line/moderate-severe: NMDA receptor antagonist **(memantine)**; ameliorates glutamate-induced cytotoxicity

COMPLICATIONS
- Death commonly results from infection, i.e. bronchopneumonia
- Haemorrhagic stroke: β-**amyloid** can deposit in cerebral blood vessels and weaken them (cerebral amyloid angiopathy)

PROGNOSIS
Average life expectancy from diagnosis is approximately 7 years (<3% survive >14 years)

ANTERIOR SPINAL ARTERY SYNDROME

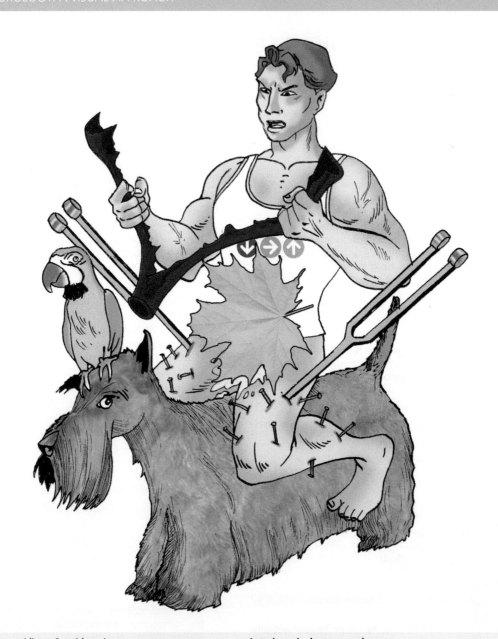

A man riding a Scottish terrier	**Anterior spinal artery syndrome** An-terrier
Covering the man's groin are leaves, similar to Adam in the Bible	**Artery of Adamkiewicz**
The man is ripping apart a large tube resembling an artery	**Aortic dissection**
His vest has three arrows pointing in different directions, arranged from left to right	**LMN lesion to UMN lesion** Down arrow = LMN lesion going to Up arrow = UMN lesion
There is a parrot sitting on top of the terrier's head	**Paraplegia**
On both the man's thighs and legs, there are multiple nails with the surrounding skin looking red	**Bilateral loss of pain and temperature** Reddened skin to signify temperature
Piercing each thigh, there is a tuning fork sticking out that is not broken	**Bilaterally intact vibration and proprioception**
There is an area of wetness around the groin	**Bladder dysfunction**

ANTERIOR SPINAL ARTERY SYNDROME

DEFINITION

A loss of bilateral corticospinal and spinothalamic function due to hypoperfusion of the anterior spinal artery

AETIOLOGY

- ASA ischaemia at the level of the spinal cord is known as anterior spinal artery syndrome (or anterior cord syndrome)
- ASA ischaemia at the level of the medulla is known as medial medullary syndrome; it has a different clinical presentation – see below
- Anatomy: the ASA supplies the anterior 2/3rd of the spinal cord and is formed by the anastomosis of the vertebral arteries at the level of the foramen magnum. As the ASA moves down, it receives 6–8 major radicular branches originating mostly from the aorta; the **artery of Adamkiewicz** (supplies ASA below ~T8) is the largest and most important of these
- Pathophysiology: the formation of the ASA from multiple sources leaves it vulnerable to watershed ischaemia, particularly during aortic occlusion or hypotension. ASA hypoperfusion leads to bilateral disruption of the corticospinal and spinothalamic tracts, with characteristic preservation of dorsal column function (as supplied by the posterior spinal arteries)
- Causes:
  - Aortic pathology: **aortic dissection**, aortic aneurysm, aortic thrombosis
  - External compression: herniated disc, neoplasm, posterior osteophyte
  - Thrombotic occlusion of the ASA

EPIDEMIOLOGY

- Spinal cord infarction accounts for approximately 1.2% of all strokes
- Annual incidence: 12/100,000

PRESENTATION

Anterior spinal artery syndrome

- Acute stage: flaccid paralysis and loss of deep tendon reflexes (**spinal shock; presents as an LMN lesion**), occurs below the level of the lesion, due to involvement of the corticospinal tract:

- Over days → weeks: evolves into spasticity and hyper-reflexia with an extensor plantar response (**UMN lesion**)
- **Paraplegia**: tetraplegia occurs if above C7
- **Bilateral loss of pain and temperature** at and below the level of injury (as is involvement of the lateral spinothalamic tracts)
- **Bilaterally intact vibratory senses, proprioception** and 2-point discrimination (intact posterior columns)
- Autonomic dysfunction: orthostatic or frank hypotension
- Sexual dysfunction, and/or bowel and **bladder dysfunction**, depending on the level of the lesion

Medial medullary syndrome

(*Added for completeness; the Investigations, Management, etc. relate to ASA syndrome.*)

- ASA infarction at the level of the medial medulla
- Clinical features are distinct from ASA syndrome due to the various ipsilateral structures affected below:
  - Medullary pyramid → contralateral hemiparesis (upper and lower limb)
  - Medial lemniscus → contralateral proprioception and vibration loss
  - Hypoglossal nerve fibres → ipsilateral tongue deviation (due to ipsilateral muscle weakness)

INVESTIGATIONS

- Best initial and most accurate test: spinal MRI; helps to confirm the underlying aetiology and rule out other causes (such as compressive myelopathy)
- Chest CT/MRI: excludes aortic dissection

MANAGEMENT

- General supportive care and rehabilitation
- Focuses on treating the primary cause of ASA insufficiency

COMPLICATIONS

Paraplegia/tetraplegia

PROGNOSIS

ASA is associated with high mortality and poor functional outcome

ATAXIA TELANGIECTASIA

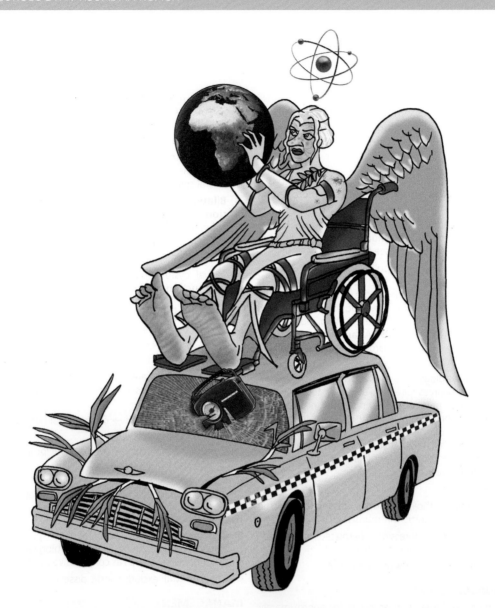

An angel is on top of a taxi	**Ataxia telangiectasia** Tel'angie' = angel
She has a spinning atom above her head	**ATM gene**
She has dilated blood vessels on her eyes, and spider naevi on her arms	**Oculocutaneous telangiectasia**
She has lots of pimples on her face, and has a large nose	**Recurrent sinopulmonary infections**
She is holding a globe with Africa shown	**↓IgA** Globe = globulin, A = Africa
The bonnet of the taxi is filled with leeks	**Leukaemia**
The angel has grey hair and wrinkled skin	**Progeric changes**
She has large feet	**↑α-fetoprotein** Alpha-'feeto'-protein, large feet as increased
There is a radio that has cracked the windscreen of the car	**Radiation**
The angel is in a wheelchair	**Wheelchair bound by age 10 years**

ATAXIA TELANGIECTASIA

DEFINITION

An autosomal recessive multisystem disorder caused by DNA repair defects, leading to progressive cerebellar ataxia and oculocutaneous telangiectasias

AETIOLOGY

- Pathophysiology: an autosomal recessive inherited mutation of the **ATM** (**A**taxia **T**elangiectasia **M**utated) gene, which normally codes for a protein kinase DNA repair enzyme that fixes double-stranded breaks in DNA. ATM mutation → inability to repair faulty genes (especially at T and B cell gene loci) → immunodeficiency and ↑risk of malignancy (leukaemia/lymphomas)
- Variant ataxia telangiectasia: a milder form of classical ataxia telangiectasia; it may reflect mutations allowing for some retained ATM protein kinase activity
- Exhibits full penetrance; sometimes it is associated with ↑rates of consanguinity

EPIDEMIOLOGY

- Incidence: ~1/100,000
- Affects ♂ and ♀ equally

PRESENTATION

- Progressive ataxia: typically presents in early childhood (1–4 y/o). Truncal ataxia precedes appendicular ataxia:
  - If ataxia develops early, it may be misdiagnosed as an ataxic variant of cerebral palsy
  - If ataxia is delayed, it may be mistaken for Friedreich's ataxia
- **Oculocutaneous telangiectasias** ('end-vessel dilation'): can be mistaken for conjunctivitis, except in ataxia telangiectasia it is dilated against white sclera. Spider naevi are also present

- Absent thymus (due to ↓T and B cells) → **recurrent infections**, particularly **sinopulmonary** (due to ↓**IgA**)
- **Leukaemia/lymphoma**: typically occurs after 10 y/o; rate of 1% a year
- **Progeric changes**: premature greying of hair, ageing changes of the skin
- Certain endocrine abnormalities (e.g. gonadal dysgenesis, testicular atrophy, diabetes mellitus)

INVESTIGATIONS

- Bloods: ↑**serum AFP** (↑ in 90%; reason unknown); **low IgA** (80%)
- **Radiation-free screening**: i.e. USS/MRI (as unable to repair DNA damage caused by X-ray/CT)
- Genetic testing: absence of **ATM protein**

MANAGEMENT

- Supportive; aim to slow/halt the neurodegeneration
- MDT approach is paramount: PT, SALT and OT
- Prompt treatment of infections; consider prophylactic antibiotics and immunisations
- Regular monitoring for malignancies; chemotherapy for associated cancers

COMPLICATIONS

- Recurrent infections
- Malignancy – usually acute lymphoblastic leukaemia (1/5 with ataxia telangiectasia)

PROGNOSIS

- Most patients are **wheelchair bound** by 10 y/o
- Many die in their 2nd decade, secondary to malignancy and respiratory failure

BROWN-SÉQUARD SYNDROME

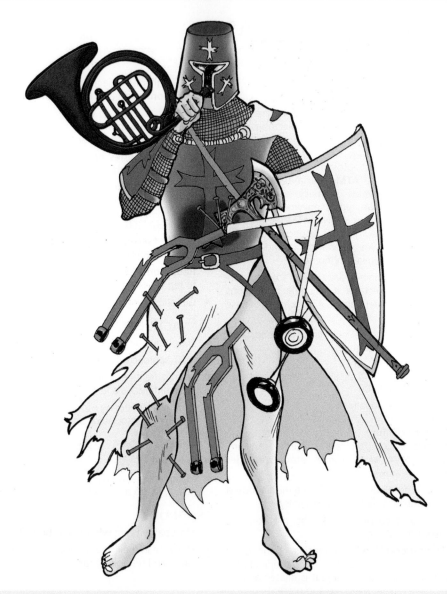

A guardian knight is in brown metal armour	**Brown-Séquard syndrome** Brown armour, Se'quard' – like 'guard'ian
On his left side, he has a large battle axe wedged into his body	**Traumatic injury; hemi-cord**
In his left hand he holds a shield with a cross symbol	**Brown-Séquard-plus syndrome**
Below the axe on the left side, his left knee is being struck by a tendon hammer. The left toes are fanned out	**Ipsilateral UMN below the lesion; hyper-reflexia, Babinski sign ipsilateral to the lesion**
At the level of the axe, there is a broken tendon hammer	**Ipsilateral LMN at the lesion site; arreflexia**
Jammed into his left leg there is broken tuning fork	**Ipsilateral vibration loss below the lesion site**
At the level of the axe on the left side, there are multiple nails and a broken tuning fork	**Ipsilateral loss of all sensation at the level of the lesion**
The knight is playing a blue French horn	**Horner's syndrome**
Below the level of the axe on the right side, there are multiple nails piercing his right leg, with redness of the skin	**Contralateral pain and temperature sensation loss below the level of the lesion** Temperature sensation loss = depicted as skin colour change

BROWN-SÉQUARD SYNDROME

DEFINITION

A syndrome caused by pathology affecting the lateral half of the spinal cord, resulting in ipsilateral loss of corticospinal tract function, touch, vibration and position sense loss and contralateral pain and temperature loss

AETIOLOGY

- Anatomy: the motor fibres of the corticospinal tracts cross at the junction of the medulla and spinal cord. The ascending dorsal column, carrying the sensations of vibration and position, runs ipsilateral and crosses above the spinal cord in the medulla. The spinothalamic tracts convey sensations of pain, temperature and crude touch from the contralateral side of the body, the fibres crossing the spinal cord upon entry from the periphery
- Pathophysiology: damage occurs to the above-mentioned ascending and descending spinal cord tracts on one-half of the spinal cord (**hemi-cord syndrome**). Scattered petechial haemorrhages develop in the grey matter (1 h post injury) and white matter (3–4 h post injury). Haemorrhagic necrosis occurs 24–36 h later
- Causes:
  - **Traumatic injury** (the most common cause): neck stab, gunshot wound or RTA
  - Non-traumatic injury: tumour, MS, disc herniation and cervical spondylosis, among others

EPIDEMIOLOGY

- The true incidence is unknown
- Average age: 40 y/o; seen ↑ in ♂ than ♀ (most likely due to ↑likelihood of traumatic injury causes)

PRESENTATION

- Most cases are partial, with varying degrees of paresis and sensory impairment
- Pure Brown-Séquard described below is rarely seen. More likely is **Brown-Séquard-plus syndrome**, which features fragments of the syndrome or additional signs and symptoms
- Ipsilateral features:
  - **Ipsilateral UMN signs below the level of the lesion; Babinski sign ipsilateral to the lesion**
  - **Ipsilateral LMN signs at the level of the lesion, i.e. arreflexia**, as the corticospinal tract decussates superiorly in the medulla
  - Ipsilateral loss of tactile, **vibration loss** and proprioception sense **below the level of the lesion**:
    - As the dorsal columns decussate superiorly in the medulla

- Fine (light) touch (dorsal column mediated) vs. crude (deep) touch (spinothalamic mediated)
  - On ipsilateral side = the dorsal column is affected, the spinothalamic tract is intact
  - Touching the patient on this side → cannot localise where they have been touched (as loss of fine touch), only that they were touched (crude touch intact)
- **Ipsilateral loss of all sensation at the level of the lesion**
- If the lesion occurs above T1, the patient may present with **Horner's syndrome**; due to damage of the ipsilateral oculosympathetic pathway
- Contralateral feature:
  - **Contralateral pain and temperature loss below the level of the lesion**: as the spinothalamic tract decussates at the level or within two segments below the lesion

INVESTIGATIONS

- Bloods: useful in non-traumatic aetiologies, i.e. infection or neoplastic. Consider LP if inflammation, e.g. if MS is suspected
- Spinal plain radiographs: for penetrating/blunt trauma to view the general extent of injury
- MRI brain and spine: checks which structures have been damaged. CT myelography (useful if MRI is C/I)

MANAGEMENT

- Acutely: C-spine immobilisation; nasogastric tube insertion if needed. Treat the underlying cause
- Medications: to treat secondary effects, such as spasticity and pain. Steroids (if spinal cord inflammation is present)
- Surgery: if due to compression from mass; surgically decompress

COMPLICATIONS

- Respiratory compromise, such as aspiration pneumonia
- Profound hypotension; 'spinal shock'
- Dysaesthesia from spinothalamic tract damage, which can be very painful

PROGNOSIS

- If the lesion is incomplete and occurs in younger patients → good prognosis
- Good prognosis for significant motor recovery

CAVERNOUS SINUS SYNDROME

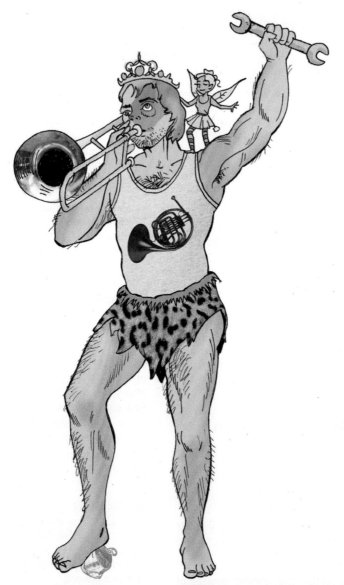

A caveman is playing the trombone	**Cavernous sinus, cavernous sinus thrombosis** Caveman = cavernous; trombone = thrombosis
He is crushing a tin can under his right foot	**Tumour (cavernous sinus)** Tin can = cancer
In his left hand he is passionately holding a spanner held in a tight fist	**Tolosa–Hunt syndrome, fistula** 'Tol'osa = tool, like spanner; fist = fistula
Sat on his left shoulder there is a fairy	**Pituitary adenoma** Pitui'tary' sounds like 'fairy'
His left eye is looking upwards, bulging and is swollen	**Ophthalmoplegia, proptosis, periorbital oedema**
He is wearing a 3-gemmed tiara	**Trigeminal nerve ($V_1 + V_2$)** 3-gem = trigeminal
The left side of his face is pink and flushed	**Hyperaesthesia (area of $V_1 + V_2$)** Pink/flushed to show the area. Normally no colour change
He is wearing a vest with a blue French horn	**Horner's syndrome**

CAVERNOUS SINUS SYNDROME

DEFINITION

A syndrome due to compression of structures within the cavernous sinus, causing multiple cranial nerve palsies

AETIOLOGY

- Anatomy/physiology: the **cavernous sinuses** are paired, venous structures located on either side of the pituitary. Blood from the eye and superficial cortex → cavernous sinus → internal jugular vein. The internal carotid artery, associated postganglionic sympathetic fibres and CN VI pass through the body of the sinus. Cranial nerves III, IV, V_1, V_2 (occasionally) pass through the lateral wall of the sinus. Compression of cavernous sinus structures can result from various pathologies, as shown below

- Causes:
  - Cavernous sinus **tumours** – most common; either primary or from nasopharyngeal tumours
  - Cavernous sinus **thrombosis** – due to spread of infection (commonly *Staphylococcus aureus*) from the frontal sinuses
    - Internal carotid artery aneurysms – painless ophthalmoplegia. Can rupture → direct C–C fistulas
- C–C **fistulas** (communication between ICA and cavernous sinus. Due to trauma/aneurysms:
  - Direct communication → abrupt presentation. Can include pulsatile proptosis
  - Indirect communication (between ICA branches and cavernous sinus) → insidious presentation
  - **Pituitary adenoma** mass effect. If large enough can cause bilateral features
  - **Tolosa–Hunt syndrome**: idiopathic granulomatous inflammation of the cavernous sinus wall. Steroid sensitive

EPIDEMIOLOGY

Incidence: 3–4/1,000,000 (intracranial venous thrombosis)

PRESENTATION

- Cavernous sinus compression features. Commonly unilateral (depending on cause):
  - CN III, IV and VI → **variable ophthalmoplegia/diplopia**; due to differing compression of each nerve
    - CN VI is generally affected before CN III/IV as it is within the sinus, adjacent to the artery

- **CN V_1** → ↓corneal sensation or **hyperaesthesia** (↑sensitivity to all sensations)
- **CN V_2** (occasionally) → ↓maxillary sensation or **hyperaesthesia** (↑sensitivity to all sensations)
- Postganglionic sympathetic fibres → **Horner's syndrome**
- Associated eye signs:
  - Pupils: may be dilated (CN III compression) or constricted (Horner's syndrome)
  - **Proptosis**: due to venous congestion
  - **Periorbital oedema**: due to venous congestion of the orbital veins
  - Painless vision loss (if the ophthalmic branch of the ICA is compromised). Occurs in severe cases
- Cavernous sinus thrombosis: headache is the most common presenting symptom. Precedes all the above features
  - Fever may also present
  - Late signs: meningism and/or sepsis

INVESTIGATIONS

- Bloods: ↑inflammatory markers (cavernous sinus thrombosis)
- LP: rules out meningitis
- MRI + gadolinium (pituitary protocol) is the most accurate test:
  - MR or CT venography are useful adjuncts
  - Consider cavernous sinus biopsy as a last resort

MANAGEMENT

- Cavernous sinus tumours: CNS tumours → chemo/radiotherapy. Pituitary tumours → dopamine agonists
- Cavernous sinus thrombosis: IV antibiotics and drainage of the primary infection site
- Cavernous sinus aneurysms: endovascular balloon occlusion
- C–C fistulas: fistula obliteration with coils

COMPLICATIONS

See Presentation

PROGNOSIS

Most cavernous lesions are treatable. Antibiotics greatly reduce the incidence and mortality from cavernous sinus thrombosis

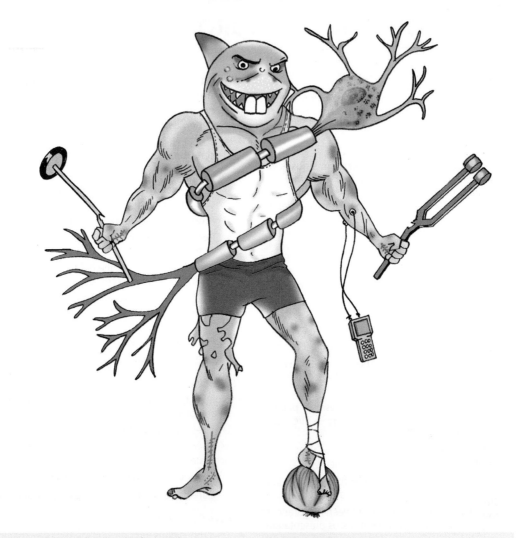

A man with a shark head has big front teeth	**Charcot–Marie–Tooth disease** Charcot = shark
Two pimples are on the side of his face	**PMP 22** PMP = pimple
He is leaning on a sliced onion-bulb	**Onion-bulb appearance**
His distal limb musculature is thinner and weaker looking than the proximal muscles	**Slowly progressive distal limb weakness**
His left foot on the onion bulb is dropped, and is bandaged	**Foot drop, ankle sprains/fractures**
His legs are shaped like inverted champagne bottles	**Inverted champagne bottles**
His right foot has a high arch	**High-arch foot**
He is holding a broken tuning fork in his left hand	**Vibration sensation lost**
He is holding a broken tendon hammer in his right hand	**Generalised arreflexia**
A large neuron is wrapped around his body	**Enlarged, palpable peripheral nerves**
A nerve conduction device is hanging from his left forearm	**Nerve conduction studies**
Surgical scars are on his hands and feet	**Hand/foot surgery**
The skin is peeling off his right thigh	**Skin breakdown**

CHARCOT–MARIE-TOOTH DISEASE

DEFINITION
A heterogeneous group of slowly progressive sensorimotor neuropathies (also known as hereditary motor and sensory neuropathy or peroneal muscular atrophy). A common cause is an alteration in the peripheral myelin protein gene

AETIOLOGY
- Pathophysiology: a hereditary defect (i.e. gene duplication) of **PMP 22** → unstable myelin sheath that is unstable and spontaneously breaks down. Schwann cells proliferate and form concentric arrays of remyelination around the demyelinated axon → results in an **onion-bulb appearance**
- CMT can be inherited autosomally or X-linked; it can also arise *de novo*. Over seven types are characterised. Only two are common to clinical practice:
  - CMT Type 1: primarily demyelinating pathology. It is the most common type; autosomal dominant
  - CMT Type 2: primarily axonal pathology. Later onset, ↓severe than Type 1

EPIDEMIOLOGY
- CMT is the most common inherited neuromuscular disorder; it affects 1/2500
- Onset: CMT Type 1 is in the 1st decade

PRESENTATION
- **Slowly progressive weakness beginning in the distal limb muscles:**
  - Leg weakness: difficulty walking and frequent tripping:
    - As weakness ↑ in severity → **foot drop**. Leads to high-stepping gait and stamping (loss of proprioception)
    - **Inverted champagne bottle,** due to the pattern of distal wasting in the legs compared to the calves
    - Intrinsic foot muscle weakness = **pes cavus (high-arch foot)**
  - Hand weakness: particularly lumbricals; poor finger control and difficulty using zippers and buttons
- Sensory loss: touch and **vibration sensation** are **lost**, beginning distally:
  - Pain and temperature sense are not affected, as these are carried by unmyelinated C fibres
- **Generalised arreflexia**
- Spinal deformities: thoracic scoliosis
- **Peripheral nerves may be palpably enlarged** (e.g. lateral popliteal nerve)

INVESTIGATIONS
- Bloods: exclude other causes of neuropathy; B$_{12}$, ANA
- **Nerve conduction studies**: velocity <38 m/s in the upper limb motor nerves
- Peripheral nerve USS of large nerves (i.e. median nerve)
- Genetic testing: PMP–22 gene duplication (seen in CMT Type 1a)
- Nerve biopsy; rarely done. Onion-bulb formation (concentric hypertrophy of the lamellar sheaths) is seen

MANAGEMENT
- No curative treatment; symptomatic only
- MDT approach: neurologist, PT, OT (rehabilitation)
- **Surgery: for hand/foot deformities**, scoliosis
- Genetic counselling

COMPLICATIONS
- **Skin breakdown/burns**: as protective sensation is usually lost distally in all four limbs
- **Ankle sprains/fractures**

PROGNOSIS
- Normal lifespan
- Usually relatively mild disability

CLUSTER HEADACHE

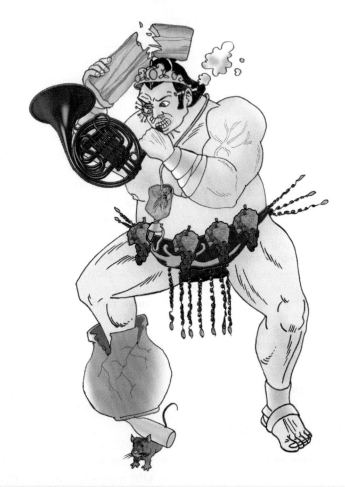

A man has multiple clusters of grapes hanging from the waist	**Cluster headache**
His foot is inside a cracked pot, that is falling over an alcohol bottle, and there is a burning cigarette over his left ear	**Hypothalamus dysfunction, alcohol, smoking** Hy-pot-halamus = pot, cracked means dysfunctional
He is wearing a 3-gemmed tiara	**Trigeminal nerve nucleus**
The man has severe redness (pain) around the right eye with needles and is in visible pain	**Males, periorbital headache, sharp pain** Pinkish hue to skin around the eye = signifies pain, not actually how the skin appears
The right eye also has associated tearing, red eye and eyelid swelling	**Ipsilateral lacrimation, conjunctival injection, eyelid oedema**
He is playing a blue French horn	**Horner's syndrome** Blue French horn – symbol for Horner
His right nostril is plugged with tissue; the left nostril is runny	**Nasal stuffiness, rhinorrhoea**
He is breaking a plank of wood over his head	**Bang head on walls/surfaces**
Around the neck he has an aeroplane oxygen mask	**High-flow oxygen**
The man is a sumo wrestler tripping over a bottle	**Sumatriptan**
Under the alcohol bottle, there is a rat whose body is squashed	**Verapamil** Ve-'rat': rat
The sumo wrestler's biceps are very muscular	**Steroids (prednisolone)**

CLUSTER HEADACHE

DEFINITION
Severe, unilateral periorbital pain that typically occurs in clusters, lasting weeks to months at a time

AETIOLOGY
- Also known as periodic migrainous neuralgia. It is distinct from migraine as it has additional ipsilateral autonomic features
- Pathophysiology: poorly understood; it is likely that due to the circadian nature of attacks, the cause is **hypothalamus dysfunction** → disinhibition of **the trigeminal nerve nucleus** → ↑sensitivity and firing with associated tearing (due to the close proximity of the greater petrosal nerve that innervates the lacrimal gland)
- Risk factors: **smoking**, **alcohol** and family history (1/20 of patients with cluster headache will also have another family member also with the condition)

EPIDEMIOLOGY
- Average onset: 25–50 y/o
- ♂:♀ = 5:1

PRESENTATION
- Abrupt, excruciating, unilateral **periorbital (orbital, supraorbital and/or temporal) headache**:
  - **Pain is sharp and penetrating** (not pulsatile as with migraine)
- Pattern of occurrence:
  - Typically experience attacks once or twice a day; patients can experience up to 8 attacks per day
  - Commonly occurs at the same time of day; particularly at night, 1–2 hours after falling asleep
  - Attacks of CHs: each attack can last 15 min to 3 h:
    - If episodic CH (85%): attacks can occur daily for 6 to 12 wk (so-called cluster periods), followed by periods of remission (up to 12 mo or longer)
    - If chronic CH (15%): attacks occur without significant periods of remission (up to 12 mo without remission or remission period <1 mo)

- Bouts typically occur once a year or every 2 y, often at the same time of year
- Associated symptoms:
  - Eye: **ipsilateral lacrimation, conjunctival injection, eyelid oedema and Horner's syndrome** (in a minority)
  - Nose: **nasal stuffiness** and **rhinorrhoea**
  - Facial: sweating or flushing
  - Other: restlessness or agitation; patients **may bang their head on walls** and furniture in distress; in contrast, migraine patients tend to typically be still
  - Symptoms can switch to the other side during a different cluster attack (so-called side shift) in 15% of cases

INVESTIGATIONS
- Diagnosis is clinical; patients must fulfil the International Headache Society guidelines
- CT/MRI brain: exclude a structural lesion as a potential cause

MANAGEMENT
- General: avoid smoking and alcohol (during attack series) and maintain a good sleep pattern
- Acute (abortive): **high-flow oxygen** (100% non-rebreathing) + subcutaneous **sumatriptan** + nasal lidocaine (to the affected side)
- Prophylaxis: **verapamil** (1st line), **prednisolone**; lithium (if severe)
- Invasive: LA/steroid injection around the greater occipital nerve on the affected side can abort bouts of CH

COMPLICATIONS
Untreated: depression, suicide (rare)

PROGNOSIS
- 10% of patients with episodic CH go on to develop chronic CH
- Head injury, smoking and alcohol use are associated with a worse prognosis

CREUTZFELDT–JAKOB DISEASE

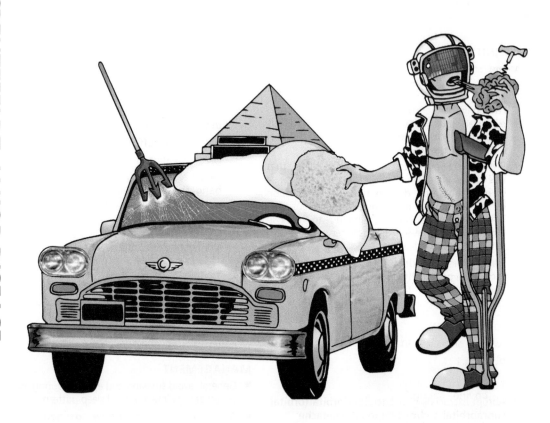

A man is leaning on a crutch	**Creutzfeldt–Jakob disease**
His helmet has prison bars on it	**Prion protein** Pri-s-on = Prion
He is washing a taxi with a large sponge	**Spongiform changes, ataxia**
He is wearing an astronaut helmet	**Astrogliosis** 'Astro'naut = 'astro'gliosis
He has an abdominal scar from an organ transplant	**Organ transplant (contaminated tissue)**
He is wearing a cow-print shirt	**Bovine spongiform encephalopathy** 'Mad cow disease'
He is eating a fresh brain	**Kuru; eating of deceased brains**
A demon trident has cracked the windscreen	**Progressive dementia**
He is wearing clown trousers and shoes	**Myoclonic jerks** Myo'clon'ic = clown
A pyramid is on top of the taxi	**Pyramidal signs on neurological examination**
He is wearing very odd clothes	**Psychiatric/behavioural changes**
A large cracked egg is on the side of the taxi	**EEG: shows characteristic changes** Egg = EEG
A corkscrew is in the brain being eaten	**Brain biopsy** Trying to remove a core of the brain

CREUTZFELDT–JAKOB DISEASE

DEFINITION

A rare, transmissible prion neurodegenerative illness

AETIOLOGY

- Pathophysiology: **PrP** exists in two forms: native, α-helical state (PrP^c) that is present in healthy neurons, which can be converted (either sporadic, inherited or transmitted) into abnormal, protease-resistant β-pleated sheet state (PrP^{sc}). This non-degradable, misfolded PrP^{sc} prion propagates refolding of native PrP^c protein into the diseased PrP^{sc} form, disrupting neuronal function and eventually causing cell death (**spongiform changes**) and **astrogliosis** (a glial response to neuronal loss and tissue damage)
- Variant CJD types:
  - Sporadic CJD: 85%; is the most common. No risk factors
  - Hereditary CJD: <15%; autosomal dominant
  - Iatrogenic CJD: prion transmission in **contaminated tissue, e.g. organ transplants** (corneal), growth hormone from cadaveric donors and blood transfusion
  - nvCJD: prion ingestion from infected cattle (**bovine spongiform encephalopathy** *aka* 'mad cow disease'); the first case appeared in 1996; earlier onset → ↑psychiatric symptoms and longer duration
  - **Kuru**: among Fore people of Papua New Guinea there was a funeral custom of ritualistic **eating of the deceased person's brain**. The practice has now ceased

EPIDEMIOLOGY

- Rare; 1/1,000,000
- Peak incidence (of sporadic): 50–70 y/o

PRESENTATION

- Neurological features: rapidly **progressive dementia**, **ataxia** and **myoclonic jerks** with **pyramidal signs**
- Initial presentation: sporadic CJD: neurological features; nvCJD: **psychiatric/behavioural changes**
- Time course: sporadic CJD: rapid, over weeks to months; nvCJD: over years

INVESTIGATIONS

- **Best initial test: EEG**; may show characteristic periodic sharp waves
- LP: 14-3-3 protein is detected in the CSF. The presence of 14-3-3 spares the need for brain biopsy
- MRI brain with diffusion-weighted imaging: shows ↑T2 and FLAIR in putamen/caudate head:
  - Pulvinar sign: the characteristic appearance of bilateral hyperintensity in the posterior nuclei of the thalamus:
    - Highly specific for the diagnosis of vCJD (in the appropriate clinical context)
- Definitive diagnosis: **brain biopsy**. Specimens must be handled carefully to avoid transmission
- Tonsil biopsy can facilitate nvCJD diagnosis

MANAGEMENT

Supportive; no effective treatment

COMPLICATIONS

Pneumonia

PROGNOSIS

Most patients die within 1 year of symptom onset

ENCEPHALITIS

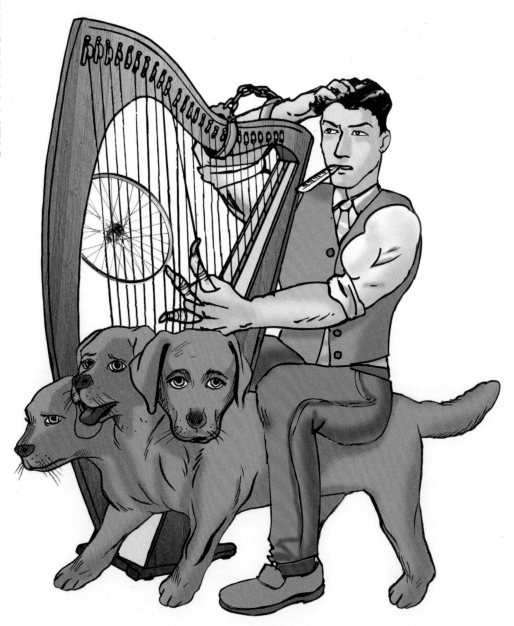

A man is handcuffed to a harp	**Encephalitis** Handcuff = 'enceph'halitis
He is trying to play the harp	**Herpes simplex virus** Harp = 'herp'es
A thermometer is in his mouth	**Fever**
He is scratching his head	**Confusion**
He is plucking the harp strings with tempura	**Temporal lobe**
He is on Cerberus, the 3-headed mythical dog	**Cerebral oedema**
There is a bicycle wheel trapped in the harp; the man has big, strong arms	**Acyclovir, steroids** A cycle wheel = acyclovir

ENCEPHALITIS

DEFINITION
Brain parenchyma inflammation, usually due to viral infection. Subsequent inflammation of the lepto-meninges is called meningoencephalitis

AETIOLOGY
- Pathophysiology: viral replication outside the CNS → reaches the brain by haematogenous spread or along neural pathways (direct invasion; seen in HSV-1). Particularly with HSV encephalitis, infection involves lymphocytic and plasma cell reaction → an acute, necrotising, asymmetrical haemorrhagic process affecting the temporal and inferior frontal lobes
- Causes: identified in only 40–70% of cases. When the cause is identified, viral infection is the most common:
- Viral: HSV, VZV, EBV, enteroviruses, CMV, West Nile virus, HIV, mumps, measles, rabies, polio:
  - **HSV-1** is responsible for 95% of cases, and causes the most severe form of encephalitis
- Bacteria: *Listeria monocytogenes*, *Mycobacteria*, spirochaetes (Lyme, syphilis)
- Parasites: protozoa (e.g. *Toxoplasma*) and helminths (rare)
- Fungi: e.g. *Cryptococcus*
- Post-infectious: e.g. ADEM
- Autoimmune/paraneoplastic: association with antibodies, e.g. anti-NMDA or anti-VGKC

EPIDEMIOLOGY
- Incidence: 7.4/100,000
- Children and the elderly are the most vulnerable

PRESENTATION
- Predominantly acute-onset **fever** with **confusion** (develops later)
- If headaches, photophobia and meningeal signs are present = meningoencephalitis
- It is important to obtain detailed sexual and travel history
- Additional clues can be obtained on examination; certain presentation features may suggest a particular diagnosis:
  - Seizures with focal neurological deficits (e.g. aphasia) → HSV encephalitis (affecting the **temporal lobes**):
    - Peripheral lesions (e.g. cold sores) have no relation to the presence of HSV encephalitis
  - Parotitis in an unvaccinated patient → mumps encephalitis
  - Flaccid paralysis that evolves into encephalitis → West Nile encephalitis
  - Hydrophobia, aerophobia, pharyngeal spasms and hyperactivity → rabies encephalitis
  - Grouped vesicles in dermatomal pattern → VZV encephalitis; absence of rash, however, does not exclude VZV as a cause

INVESTIGATIONS
- Best initial test: CT head; shows **cerebral oedema**
- Most accurate tests:
  - MRI; in HSV there is characteristic oedema of the temporal lobes; the presence of hydrocephalus may suggest a non-viral cause (e.g. bacterial, fungal or parasitic)
  - PCR of CSF (HSV, CMV, EBV, VZV)
- Blood: ↑lymphocytes (as viral), viral serology
- CSF: lymphocytosis, ↑protein and normal glucose (similar to viral meningitis), viral PCR:
  - Presence of RBCs in CSF without a history of trauma → HSV encephalitis
- EEG: periodic high-voltage sharp waves and slow-wave complexes at 2–3 second intervals in the temporal leads
- HIV testing: recommended in all individuals with possible encephalitis

MANAGEMENT
- Consider admission to ITU if there is significant deterioration. Monitor vital signs carefully
- Start empirical IV **acyclovir** +/- antibiotics (↓mortality rate from 70% to 25%). If acyclovir resistant, consider foscarnet
- **+/- steroids** (e.g. dexamethasone, depending on whether **cerebral oedema** is present or not)
- Consider anticonvulsants, depending on presentation

COMPLICATIONS
Epilepsy, cognitive impairment

PROGNOSIS
- HSV encephalitis is associated with high mortality (fatal if untreated and causes death in 7–10 days):
  - Even with optimal treatment, mortality is 20–25%

EPILEPSY

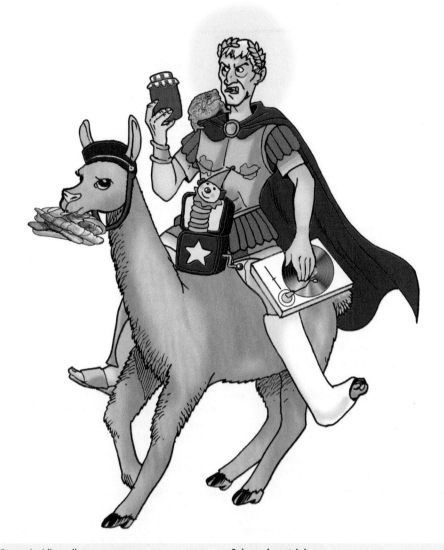

Julius Caesar is riding a llama	**Seizure, lamotrigine** Caesar = seizure; llama = lamotrigine
He has bags under his eyes	**Sleep deprivation**
He has an aura around his head	**Epileptic aura**
There is a Jack-in-the-box toy in front of him	**Jacksonian seizure**
There is a toad sitting on his right shoulder	**Todd's paresis**
The llama is eating tempura inside a bun	**Temporal lobe, carbamazepine** Bun = carbs → carbamazepine
With his left hand Julius Caesar is DJ-ing	**Déjà vu**
With right hand, he is holding a jam jar	**Jamais vu**
He is biting his tongue	**Tongue biting**
He has a wet patch in the groin area	**Urinary incontinence**
There are wet patches around his nipples due to lactation	**Prolactin**
The llama is wearing a valet's hat	**Sodium valproate**
Julius Caesar is wearing a cast on his left leg	**Fracture** (a complication)

EPILEPSY

DEFINITION

Recurrent (>2) unprovoked **seizures** (paroxysmal, synchronous cortical electrical discharges). It is a diagnosis of exclusion

AETIOLOGY

- Pathophysiology: triggers (e.g. flashing lights, **sleep deprivation**) ↑neuronal excitability (↑glutamate/↓GABA) past the seizure threshold (when cells fire uncontrollably). Epileptic individuals have ↓seizure threshold, leading to various **epileptic auras** described below, depending on the location
- Causes (mostly idiopathic):
  - Primary epilepsy syndrome: idiopathic generalised epilepsy, temporal lobe epilepsy
  - Secondary seizures: cortical lesion, pyrexia (especially in children), CNS infection, trauma, drugs (TCA, isoniazid), metabolic (uraemia, hypoglycaemia, hypo/hypernatraemia, hypo/hypercalcaemia)

EPIDEMIOLOGY

- Highest incidence: early childhood or in the elderly
- Lifetime risk: 1–2%

PRESENTATION

- Focal (partial, 50–60%): simple or complex depending on the ARAS involvement:
  - Simple (no change in consciousness):
    - Parietal lobe: vertigo, distorted body image
    - Frontal lobe: **Jacksonian seizure** (small jerking movements of the hands/face (as these regions have the largest representation in the motor cortex), **Todd's paresis** (post-ictal hemiparesis)
  - Complex (impaired consciousness):
    - **Temporal lobe**: hallucinations, lip-smacking, **déjà vu** (overfamiliarity), **jamais vu** (no familiarity)
- Generalised (40%): involves the whole brain. Initiated in deep midline brain structures (i.e. brainstem) and then projects simultaneously to both cortices:
  - Tonic–clonic: grand mal (60%): tonic, then clonic phase. 'Cry' as the diaphragm spasms and air is expelled
  - **Tongue biting, loss of bladder control**
  - Atonic: loss of muscle tone; have 'drop attacks' → fall to the floor as no postural tone

- Myoclonic: often teenagers, sporadic jerking movement, usually in the arms
- Absence (*aka* petit mal): often children, brief (~15 s) staring episodes. No ↓ in postural tone

INVESTIGATIONS

- Epilepsy is a diagnosis of exclusion; a witness account or video recording (best) is better than most tests
- Bloods: FBC, U&E, LFT, glucose, Ca^{2+}, Mg^{2+}
- CT/MRI brain: exclude space-occupying lesion
- EEG: only useful to differentiate between epileptic types, not for finding out the cause
- ↑**Prolactin**: transiently rises after a 'true' seizure; helps to distinguish from pseudo-seizures

MANAGEMENT

- Patient education: avoid triggers, have supervision for activities such as swimming, keep a seizure diary
- AED treatment – can only be started after >2 unprovoked seizures:
  - Maintain monotherapy. Medication may be stopped if the patient is seizure-free for 2 years:
    - Partial seizure: 1st line is **lamotrigine** or **carbamazepine**
    - Generalised seizure: 1st line is **sodium valproate**
- Surgery: VNS or DBS; used only for refractory cases. Surgery involves specialist epilepsy nurses in the patient's care
- Driving: inform the DVLA. Regarding Group 1 vehicles (car and motorcycle):
  - If a seizure occurs when awake → stop driving for 1 year
  - If a seizure occurs when asleep → can drive, but only if there is no awake attack for 3 years

COMPLICATIONS

- **Fracture** with tonic–clonic seizures, injuries 2° to seizures
- SUDEP
- Status epilepticus (seizure >30 min or repeated seizures with failure to regain consciousness)

PROGNOSIS

- 50% remission at 1 year
- ↓Likelihood of remission with longer persistence of seizures

EXTRADURAL HAEMATOMA

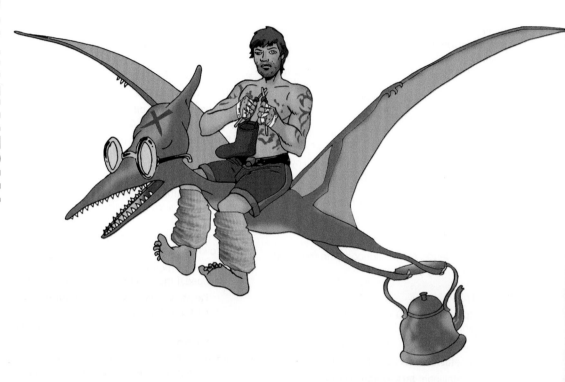

A pterodactyl has a large X on its head	**Extradural haematoma** X-tradural
A man is riding the pterodactyl	**Pterion** Pterodactyl = pterion
He looks like a mixed martial arts (MMA) fighter	**MMA**
His knuckles are bruised and bloodied	**Uncal herniation** Knuckle = uncal
He is wearing loose, baggy leg warmers	**Lucid interval** Lucid = loose
His right eye has a 'down and out' appearance. The pterodactyl is holding a kettle with its hind legs	**CN III palsy, Kernohan's notch** Kernohan = Kettle
The pterodactyl has biconvex-shaped glasses	**Biconvex lentiform collection**
The man is knitting a small red sock	**Suture lines**
Both his feet are fanning upwards	**Bilateral Babinksi sign +ve**

EXTRADURAL HAEMATOMA

DEFINITION

Traumatic accumulation of blood between the dura mater and the skull (inner table)

AETIOLOGY

- Traumatic injury to the head, e.g. RTA or focused blow
- Pathophysiology (seen in 85% of cases): **pterion fracture** → rupture of **MMA** → rapid expansion under systemic arterial pressure within the dural space (between the periosteal dural layer and the meningeal dural layer). If large enough → risk of herniation (usually **uncal**). Remainder of cases are due to bleeding from middle meningeal veins, dural sinus or bone/diploic veins
- 20% are associated with acute subdural haematoma

EPIDEMIOLOGY

- 1% of head trauma admissions
- Mainly young adults. It is rare at the extremes of age (as dura ↑adherent to the skull at these ages)

PRESENTATION

- Classical sequelae (<30% of cases):
  - Head trauma; initially unconscious due to concussion:
  - Followed by recovery and a **lucid interval** (minutes to hours) where the haematoma sub-clinically expands:
    - Approximately one-third of have a characteristic lucid interval
  - Neurological deterioration (↓GCS); including evidence of herniation:
    - Ipsilateral pupillary dilatation: due to ↑ICP → compression, causing **CN III palsy**
    - Contralateral hemiparesis: due to compression of the ipsilateral cerebral peduncle
    - Ipsilateral hemiparesis: can occur as a 'false localising sign' due to compression of the contralateral cerebral peduncle against the tentorial edge (so-called **Kernohan notch** phenomenon)

- Later stages due to progression and herniation:
  - Coma and decerebrate rigidity
  - Cushing response (hypertension, bradycardia and respiratory irregularity) → death
  - Deterioration usually occurs over a 'few' hours; however, extradural haematoma formation in the posterior fossa can produce a very rapid deterioration to death, measured in minutes
- Associated: headache, vomiting and seizures

INVESTIGATIONS

- Plain skull X-ray: may see a skull fracture
- CT head: a **biconvex (lentiform)**, hyperdense blood collection may be seen. The collection **does not cross suture lines** (the dura is attached more firmly to the skull here; hence the lentiform shape):
  - Possible midline shift with ↑severity
- CT cervical spine: excludes any associated neck injury

MANAGEMENT

- Resuscitation if needed
- Emergency neurosurgical evacuation (open craniotomy and haematoma evacuation)

COMPLICATIONS

- Permanent neurological deficits
- Post-traumatic seizures may develop 1–3 months post injury (due to cortical damage); risk ↓ with time
- Death; respiratory arrest from **uncal herniation**

PROGNOSIS

- 5–10% mortality with optimal treatment. Mortality ↑ with delayed treatment
- Underlying brain parenchyma is relatively intact if treated promptly
- There is a worse prognosis if the patient is **bilaterally Babinski sign +ve** or has decerebration pre-operation

FACIAL NERVE PALSY

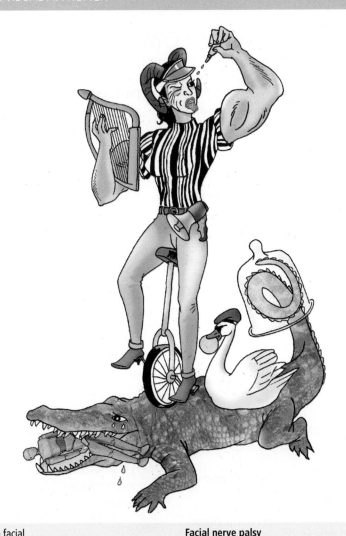

The woman has a facial	**Facial nerve palsy**
She is trying to raise her eyebrows, smile and close her eyes. The left side of her face is expressionless	**LMN palsy:** absent forehead crease, inability to close the eye, droopy smile
She has a loudspeaker attached to her waist	**Hyperacusis**
She is wearing a stripy top, and her tongue is pale and cracked	**Stroke, dry mouth, impairment of taste** Stripe = stroke; cracked tongue = dry mouth; pale tongue = bland/tasteless
A swan is on a crocodile and is wearing a green beret and has a lime slice in its mouth	**Acoustic neuroma, GBS, Lyme disease** Swan = schwannoma; green beret = Guillain–Barré
The woman is wearing a visor hat, and has ram-like horns coming out of her head	**Myasthenia gravis, Ramsay Hunt syndrome** Myasthenia gra-'vis'-or
The crocodile's tail is curled up inside a bell jar	**Bell's palsy**
The woman is playing a small harp with her right hand	**HSV**
The crocodile has broken a male crash-dummy doll into two	**House–Brackmann** Break-man
With her left hand, the woman is squirting eye drops into her left eye. She has large biceps	**Artificial tears/eye lubricant, prednisolone** Biceps = steroids = prednisolone
The woman is riding a unicycle on top of the crying crocodile	**Acyclovir, crocodile tear syndrome** 'Acicl'ovir = unicycle

FACIAL NERVE PALSY

DEFINITION

A central or peripheral CN VII lesion causing a clinical syndrome with characteristic facial muscle weakness

AETIOLOGY

- Anatomy/pathophysiology: the facial nerve is a mixed nerve: 'face, ear, taste, tear'. (→ = pathology due to palsy):
  - Motor innervation (supplies all facial expression muscles); of importance:
    - Frontalis (raises the forehead), orbicularis oculi (closes the eyelids) and orbicularis oris (closes the mouth):
      - ‡ UMN lesion (damage to motor cortex or the connection between the cortex and facial nucleus [corticobulbar tract]) → orbicularis oculi and frontalis are spared (due to bilateral UMN innervation); contralateral orbicularis oris has spastic paralysis:
        - » Presents as a contralateral droopy smile with forehead sparing
      - ‡ **LMN** lesion (damage to facial nucleus and/or its outflow) → ipsilateral flaccid paralysis of the frontalis, orbicularis oculi and orbicularis oris:
        - » Presents as **absent forehead crease, inability to close the eye and a droopy smile**
        - » Bell's phenomenon: the eyeball normally rolls up when the eyelid is closed (protective mechanism). If there is an LMN lesion, the patient cannot close the orbicularis oculi → eyeball rolls up but the eyelid remains open
    - Stapedius (via nerve to stapedius) → **hyperacusis**:
      - ‡ Acts to contract the stapedius to ↓stapes bone movement to dampen sound. Palsy → ↑stapes movement
  - Parasympathetic innervation:
    - Lacrimal secretion → dry eyes. Worsened in an LMN lesion as the orbicularis oculi cannot close the eye
      - ‡ Occasionally can develop ↑tearing; *see Complications*
    - Submandibular + sublingual salivary gland secretion (via chorda tympani nerve) → **dry mouth**
  - Sensory innervation:
    - Taste from anterior 2/3rd of the tongue (via chorda tympani nerve) → **impairment of taste**
    - Retro-auricular (behind the ear) sensation → post-auricular anaesthesia
    - Part of tympanic membrane sensation → partial tympanic membrane anaesthesia

- Causes:
  - Central (UMN) lesion: **stroke**, brain tumour, MS
  - Peripheral (LMN) lesion: otitis media, **acoustic neuroma**, parotid tumour, diabetes
    - Bilateral palsy: consider sarcoidosis**, GBS, Lyme disease** (can also cause unilateral palsy):
      - ‡ Must rule out **myasthenia gravis** as it mimics facial nerve palsy
    - **Ramsay Hunt syndrome**: VZV reactivation in the geniculate ganglion of CN VII:
      - ‡ Facial nerve palsy + auricular vesicular rash. Hearing loss + tinnitus (as CN VIII is in close proximity to the geniculate ganglion)
    - **Bell's palsy**: acute, isolated, idiopathic, LMN palsy thought secondary to **HSV** infection. Diagnosis is one of exclusion and is the commonest cause of isolated LMN facial weakness
- Severity: graded by **House–Brackmann Facial Nerve Grading System** (1: normal power, 6: total paralysis)

EPIDEMIOLOGY

- Bell's palsy: annual incidence is 30/100,000
- Most cases are 20–50 y/o

PRESENTATION

See Aetiology

INVESTIGATIONS

- CT/MRI brain: rule in/out the various causes
- Serology: Lyme disease, HSV, VZV

MANAGEMENT

- Cause dependent. General: protect the eyes; consider using an eye patch and **artificial tears/eye lubricant** to protect the cornea
- Ramsay Hunt syndrome: oral **acyclovir**
- Bell's palsy: high-dose **prednisolone** is given <72 h of onset (only if Ramsay Hunt is excluded). There is little evidence for the efficacy of acyclovir use

COMPLICATIONS

- Corneal abrasion/ulceration
- **Crocodile tear syndrome**: rare, during LMN palsy recovery → aberrant growth of nerve fibres to the superior salivatory nucleus connects to the lacrimal gland. When the patient salivates (eating food) → causes crying (recall normally LMN damage → ↓tearing)

PROGNOSIS

In Bell's palsy recovery begins by 2 weeks; 85% fully recover over time but 10% have residual weakness

FRIEDREICH'S ATAXIA

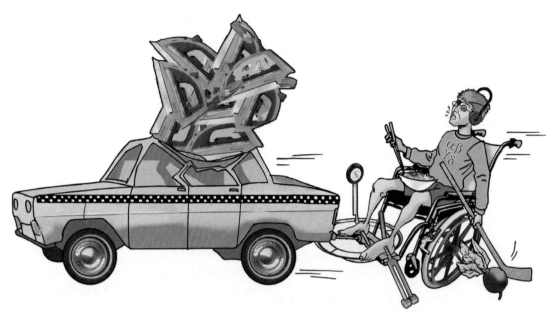

A young boy is carrying a bowl of fried rice and wearing a Greek fraternity top	**Friedreich's ataxia, frataxin** Fried rice = Friedreich; 'frat'ernity = *Frataxin*
A taxi is crushed by a huge ball made up of compressed irons	**Ataxia, iron accumulation**
The boy is gargling water in his mouth	**GAA triplet repeats** 'GAA-rgle'
There is a broken tendon hammer through his right ankle	**Absent ankle jerks**
There is a broken tuning fork through his left ankle	**Vibration sensory loss**
His legs are very thin	**Ascending muscle weakness**
He is wearing noise-cancelling headphones	**Hearing loss**
He has an eye patch making it difficult to see	**Visual disturbance**
Both his feet have a high arch. Underneath his right foot there is a dinner plate	**High foot arch, high-arched palate** Plate = palate
He has a hockey stick, and has hit a beetroot	**HCM, diabetes** Hockey = H'o'CM; Dia'beet'es
He is confined to a wheelchair	**Wheelchair bound**

FRIEDREICH'S ATAXIA

DEFINITION

An autosomal recessive GAA triplet repeat expansion disorder affecting multiple myelinated tracts and myocardial tissue

AETIOLOGY

- Pathophysiology: **frataxin** (a gene on chr. 9) is essential for mitochondrial iron regulation and prevention of reactive oxygen species formation. Frataxin mutation leads to **iron accumulation** → oxidative damage → degeneration of multiple myelinated tracts (posterior columns, corticospinal, spinocerebellar tracts and cerebellum). Sensory neurons involving proprioception are affected early in the disease, hence **ataxia** is an early feature
- 98% of patients have **GAA triplet repeat**; the size of the expansion correlates with disease severity
- Does not lead to anticipation, unlike other trinucleotide repeat disorders

EPIDEMIOLOGY

- It is the most common inherited ataxia in the UK
- ♂ and ♀ are equally affected
- Onset: 10–15 y/o (late onset is possible up to 50 y/o)
- Prevalence: 1.8/100,000

PRESENTATION

- Neurological features:
  - Progressive ataxia of all four limbs and gait is the usual presenting symptom:
    - Mainly from dorsal root ganglia degeneration → sensory ataxia
  - **Absent ankle jerks**/extensor plantars (seen in 90% of patients)
  - Cerebellar dysarthria (may begin >5 years after onset)
  - Ascending proprioception and **vibration sensory loss**
  - **Ascending muscle weakness**: involving feet and legs (88%); followed later by hand and arm weakness
  - **Hearing loss/visual disturbance**: optic atrophy or nystagmus are common
  - Bladder dysfunction with urinary urgency and later onset of incontinence (25–50%)
- Associated features (may precede neurological symptoms by several years):

- **High-arched palate and feet** (pes cavus)
- Scoliosis
- HCM:
  - 75% of patients develop left ventricular hypertrophy
  - 10% of patients develop conduction abnormalities
  - However, cardiac symptoms are relatively rare and occur later in disease
- Diabetes mellitus
- Peripheral cyanosis, oedema and cold feet: due to reduced muscle activity

INVESTIGATIONS

- Echo: for **HCM**
- MRI brain and spinal cord: for cervical spinal cord atrophy; no cerebellar atrophy is seen:
  - If cerebellar atrophy is present, consider an alternative hereditary ataxia other than Freidreich's ataxia
- Nerve conduction studies: absent sensory action potentials in 90%
- Brainstem auditory evoked response/visual evoked potentials: may be abnormal
- Genetic analysis

MANAGEMENT

- Supportive with MDT approach: Neurologist, Geneticist, PT, SALT, OT +/- cardiology, orthopaedics (regarding complications/other features)
- Annual review: neurological, musculoskeletal and cardiac assessment
- Medical: most RCTs focus on antioxidant therapy. At present, none show significant benefit
- Surgery: for scoliosis, pes cavus

COMPLICATIONS

- **HCM** (90%; the most common cause of death)
- **Diabetes mellitus** (10–20%)
- Optic atrophy (25–-50%)

PROGNOSIS

- **Wheelchair bound** a few years after diagnosis
- Average life expectancy: 40–50 y/o

FRONTOTEMPORAL DEMENTIA

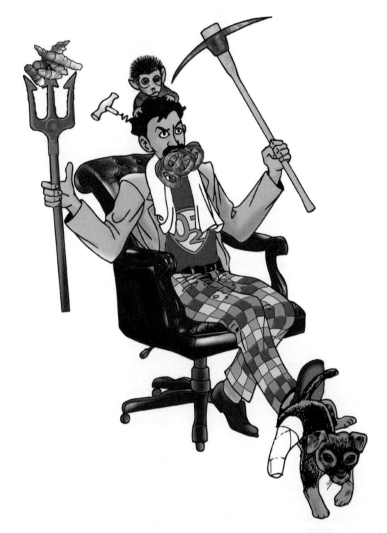

A businessman is holding a big pickaxe in one hand and a demon trident in the other	**Pick's disease (frontotemporal dementia subtype)**
He is wearing a towel around his neck	**Tau protein** Tau = towel
Tempura is attached to the ends of the demon trident	**Temporal lobe**
He is wearing a T-shirt with an O2- logo	**MND (superoxide dismutase)** *(see Motor neuron disease chapter for more information)*
He is wearing very odd clothes	**Socially inappropriate behaviour** Clothing is socially inappropriate for a businessman
A wet patch is noted around the groin area	**Public urination**
He has lots of pretzels shoved in his mouth	**Witzelsucht, hyperorality** 'Witzel'sucht = pretzel
He is kicking an injured puppy	**Empathy loss**
He is sitting in an executive chair	**Executive dysfunction**
There is a small monkey on top of his head	**Primitive reflexes** Primate = primitive
There is a corkscrew lodged in the man's head	**Brain biopsy**

FRONTOTEMPORAL DEMENTIA

DEFINITION

A rare, progressive degenerative disorder, characterised by selective frontal and temporal lobe atrophy

AETIOLOGY

- Pathophysiology: **tau** is a microtubule-associated protein that stabilises neuronal structure. Defects (sporadic or genetic) → poorly understood mechanism leading to frontal/**temporal** cortical neuron degeneration
- FTD is an umbrella term for several clinical presentations (90% sporadic, 10% genetic):
  - Behavioural variant:
    - Most common clinical subtype (*see Presentation*)
    - Historically known as **Pick's disease**; hence Pick's disease ≠ FTD, rather it is a subtype of FTD
    - Can sometimes coexist with **MND** (may precede or follow FTD development)
  - PPA: prominent decline in language ability; three variants:
    - Non-fluent PPA: laboured articulation/speech, anomia, word-finding deficit
    - Semantic PPA: impaired single-word comprehension and object naming (e.g. 'animal' for 'dog')
    - Logopenic PPA: impaired single-word retrieval and repetition. Preserved single-word comprehension

EPIDEMIOLOGY

- <5% of all dementias
- Commonly present at 60 y/o+

PRESENTATION

- Gradual, insidious progression
- Behavioural variant FTD (2/3rd of FTD cases). Early behavioural/personality changes:
  - International Behavioural Variant FTD Criteria (2011). Diagnosis requires 3/6 features (below)
    - 1 Behavioural disinhibition:
      - **Socially inappropriate behaviour** (e.g. kissing strangers, **public urination**)
      - **Witzelsucht**: compulsive telling of inappropriate jokes/puns
    - 2 Apathy/inertia
    - 3 Sympathy/**empathy loss**
    - 4 Repetitive, compulsive behaviour

- 5 **Hyperorality** and dietary changes:
  - Oral exploration of inedible objects
  - Altered food preferences, e.g. carbohydrate cravings
- 6 Executive dysfunction:
  - Difficulty with planning and organisation (**executive skills**)
  - Relative sparing of memory, cognition and visuospatial skills; initially patients perform well on the MMSE as it does not assess behaviour and judgement
- Later stages: neurological exam displays **primitive reflexes** (palmo-mental, grasp, pout reflexes)

INVESTIGATIONS

- Bloods: dementia screen; B_{12}, U&E, TFTs, ANA, syphilis serology (if appropriate)
- CT/MRI head: shows circumscribed frontal/**temporal lobe** atrophy (unilateral or bilateral)
- LP: CSF biomarkers; in AD see ↑phosphorylated tau protein, ↓β-amyloid. These help to distinguish from FTD
- **Brain biopsy**: in very select patients → may display Pick bodies (cytoplasmic inclusions of tau fibrils)

MANAGEMENT

- No cure; largely supportive
- MDT approach is paramount; supportive therapy is provided for patients and their family
- Treatment of associated symptoms: depression, agitation and sleep disturbances
- Pharmacological management; although AD and FTD share similar features, cholinergic neurons are not affected, hence drugs are unable to promote symptomatic improvement in FTD
- Disinhibition and compulsive behaviours: SSRIs (evidence is limited)
- Agitation/psychosis: atypical antipsychotics can be helpful

COMPLICATIONS

Financial/legal crisis

PROGNOSIS

- Increasing disability
- Average survival 8–10 years
- The worst prognosis is when FTD is overlapped with **MND** (survival 3–5 years)

GUILLAIN–BARRÉ SYNDROME

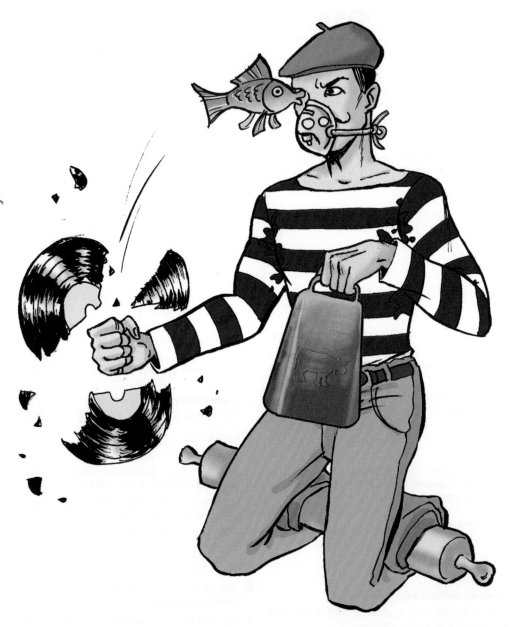

A Frenchman is wearing a green beret	**Guillain–Barré syndrome** Green beret = Guillain–Barré
He is holding a cowbell in his left hand	***Campylobacter jejuni*** 'Cowbell' sounded out loosely sounds like *Campylobacter*
A fish is attached to his right eye	**Miller Fisher syndrome**
His legs are wound around a rolling pin and moving up	**Symmetrical ascending lower limb weakness**
He has profuse sweating under his armpits	**Autonomic dysfunction**
He is wearing an oxygen mask	**Respiratory compromise**
A vinyl album disc is being crushed with his right hand	**Albuminocytological dissociation** Album = albuminocytological; disc = dissociation

GUILLAIN–BARRÉ SYNDROME

DEFINITION

A heterogeneous inflammatory condition causing demyelination and axonal degeneration, resulting in acute, ascending, progressive neuropathy

AETIOLOGY

- Pathophysiology: autoimmune attack due to molecular mimicry between antibodies created from a recent infection → cross-react and target antigens on peripheral nerve myelin (i.e. gangliosides and glycolipids) covering the spinal roots and peripheral nerves (cranial nerves may be involved) → ↓nerve conduction → flaccid paralysis
- Usually develops 3–4 weeks following a respiratory/GI infection (75% of cases):
  - **Campylobacter jejuni** (most common cause): ↑virulence as has antigens in its capsule that are similar to myelin
  - CMV (second most common cause), EBV, HBV, HZV and mycoplasma. HIV is also implicated
- GBS variants: historically it was considered a single disorder, but is now recognised as an umbrella term with several variants:
  - AIDP: most common clinically; 85–90% of cases (see Presentation)
  - AMAN: purely motor, ↑prevalence in children
  - AMSAN: severe form of AMAN, sensory nerves are affected
  - **Miller Fisher syndrome:**
    - A rare triad of ophthalmoplegia, ataxia and arreflexia. It is seen in 5% of all GBS cases
    - Usually presents as descending paralysis rather than ascending, as seen in other GBS variants
    - Antibodies against GQ1b (ganglioside component of nerve) is present in 85–90% of cases
  - Acute panautonomic neuropathy: rare; involves sympathetic and parasympathetic nervous systems
  - Pure sensory GBS: sensory loss, sensory ataxia and arreflexia in a symmetrical and widespread pattern
  - Pharyngeal–cervical–brachial weakness: oropharyngeal, neck and shoulder muscle weakness

EPIDEMIOLOGY

- Incidence: 1–2 per 100,000/year
- ↑Incidence in ♂
- Peak ages are 15–35 y/o and 50–75 y/o

PRESENTATION

- Subacute (over days to weeks) **symmetrical ascending muscle weakness** (lower to upper) with arreflexia
- Ascending sensory dysfunction: loss of proprioception, paraesthesia
- **Autonomic dysfunction**: arrhythmias, postural hypotension
- Can ascend to involve the diaphragm (causing **respiratory compromise**) and cranial nerves (facial weakness is common)
- Pain in the lower back is often the first symptom (due to inflammatory damage to spinal nerve roots)

INVESTIGATIONS

- GBS is mainly a clinical diagnosis
- Best initial test: LP; shows **albuminocytological dissociation** (↑CSF protein, normal WCC):
  - Present in 50–66% of patient in the first week after symptom onset, and >75% in the third week
  - Hence better to perform LP ~2 weeks after symptom onset
- Most accurate test: nerve conduction studies (↓conduction velocity due to peripheral nerve demyelination)
- Spirometry: measure FVC; major determinant for the need to admit the patient to ITU
- ECG: arrhythmias, i.e. 2nd/3rd degree AV block, T-wave abnormalities, etc

MANAGEMENT

- IVIG or plasmapheresis (steroids are not indicated and may delay recovery)
- Monitor FVC 4-hourly (for respiratory compromise) and ECG (for arrhythmias)
- May require ITU admission for respiratory assistance

COMPLICATIONS

- Respiratory failure
- Cardiac arrhythmias

PROGNOSIS

- 85% make a complete recovery in 3–6 months
- <5% mortality

HORNER'S SYNDROME

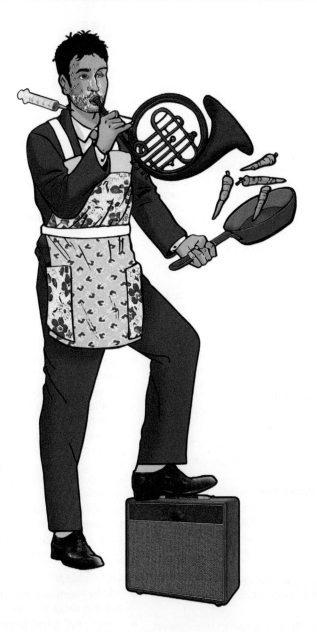

A man in a suit is playing a blue French horn	**Horner's syndrome**
A syringe is stabbed into the side of his neck	**Syringomyelia, neck trauma/surgery**
He is flipping carrots in a frying pan	**ICA dissection, Pancoast tumour** Pan = Pancoast, Carrot = Internal 'Carot'id
The left side of his face is has a droopy eyelid, small pupil and dry face (no sweating)	**Ptosis, miosis, anihidrosis**
The left eye iris colour is different from the right	**Iris heterochromia**
There is cocaine powder around the sides of his nose	**Cocaine test**
He is wearing a flowery apron	**Apraclonidine test** Apra = apron
His right foot is resting on a portable amplifier	**Hydroxyamphetamine** 'Amp'lifier = hydroxy'amp'hetamine

HORNER'S SYNDROME

DEFINITION

An interrupted ipsilateral sympathetic innervation (3-neuron oculosympathetic pathway) to the head, eye and neck

AETIOLOGY

- It is characterised by which order neuron is affected:
  - 1st order neuron (central lesion). From hypothalamus → lateral horn of T1:
    - MS, **syringomyelia**, intracranial tumours, Wallenberg syndrome
  - 2nd order neuron (preganglionic lesion). From lateral horn of T1 → cervical sympathetic chain:
    - **Neck trauma/surgery**, **Pancoast tumour**, cervical rib, neuroblastoma, thyroidectomy
  - 3rd order neuron (postganglionic lesion). From cervical sympathetic chain → neurons diverge and take two paths: those to the pupil and eyelid muscle travel along the ICA through the cavernous sinus to reach the orbit; those to the facial sweat glands travel with the external carotid artery to the face:
    - Cavernous sinus thrombosis, **ICA dissection**, carotid aneurysm, CH

EPIDEMIOLOGY

There are no epidemiological data on Horner's syndrome in adults

PRESENTATION

- **Partial ptosis**: Müller's muscle denervation – the small eyelid muscle that assists in upper lid elevation:
  - Levator palpebrae superiosis muscle is unaffected, hence ptosis is not as marked
- **Miosis**: dilator pupillae denervation. Degree of anisocoria is ↑ in the dark compared with in the light
- Hemifacial **anhidrosis**: sweat gland denervation. Anhidrosis determines the site of the lesion:
  - Head, arms and trunk → central lesion
  - Face only → preganglionic lesion
  - No anhidrosis/limited to the middle part of the forehead → postganglionic lesion; as facial sweat gland innervation is unaffected by ICA pathology
- Apparent enophthalmos (due to partial ptosis, gives the eye a sunken appearance)
- Facial flushing: if a preganglionic lesion
- Orbital pain/headache: if a postganglionic lesion

- Congenital Horner's: all features, including **iris heterochromia**:
  - The affected eye is hypopigmented (i.e. blue). Iris pigmentation is under sympathetic control prior to 2 y/o, hence disruption leads to the default blue colour
- Possible associated neurological symptoms; these are helpful to localise the lesion:
  - Diplopia, vertigo, ataxia → brainstem
  - Bilateral/ipsilateral weakness, sensory, bladder or bowel dysfunction → spinal cord
  - Arm pain/hand weakness → brachial plexus/lung apex
  - CN VI palsy → cavernous sinus
  - Head and neck pain → carotid artery

INVESTIGATIONS

- To exclude other causes:
  - CT/MRI (intracranial mass), angiography (carotid artery dissection), CXR (Pancoast tumour)
- To classically confirm Horner's: **cocaine** eye drops test. Cocaine blocks NA uptake → ↑NA in synaptic cleft:
  - Cocaine in normal pupil: sympathetic pathway intact → pupil dilation
  - Cocaine in Horner's pupil: sympathetic denervation → cocaine cannot ↑NA → no pupil dilation
- Cocaine has been replaced by apraclonidine; weak α-agonist (mimics NA):
  - **Apraclonidine** in normal pupil: sympathetic pathway intact → no denervation supersensitivity → no pupil dilation
  - **Apraclonidine** in Horner's pupil: denervation supersensitivity leads to α1-receptor upregulation on dilator pupillae → marked pupil dilation
- To localise lesion (if 1st, 2nd or 3rd order): **hydroxyamphetamine** (simulates NA release from 3rd order neuron):
  - In normal pupil: 3rd order neuron intact → ↑NA release → pupil dilation
  - Horner's pupil: give hydroxyamphetamine. If pupil dilation → 3rd order neuron intact (hence 1st/2nd order neuron problem). If no dilation, lesion is at a 3rd order neuron

MANAGEMENT, COMPLICATIONS AND PROGNOSIS

Horner' syndrome is a physical sign. Management, complications and prognosis are dependent on managing the underlying cause

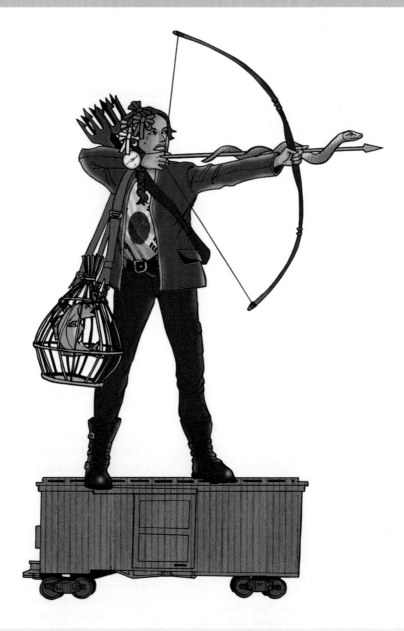

A girl is dressed in hunting attire	**Huntington's disease**
She is wearing 4 ribbons in her hair	**Tetrabenazine, chr. 4** Tetra = 4; 'ribbon' = tet'raben'azine
She is holding a cage, which has a cod fish inside	**CAG repeats, caudate nucleus** Cage = CAG Cod = caudate
She is biting her lip, as if anticipating something	**Anticipation**
She is wearing a wrist compass, pointing west	**Westphal variant**
Demon tridents are in her arrow bag	**Dementia**
The South Korean flag is on her T-shirt	**Chorea**
She is crying because she is sad	**Depression**
She is standing on top of a box-car	**Box-car ventricles**
A serpent is wound around her arrow	**Reserpine**

HUNTINGTON'S DISEASE

DEFINITION

A hyperkinetic, autosomal dominant neurodegenerative disorder due to triplet repeat (CAG) expansions in the gene coding for huntingtin protein on **chr. 4**. It is characterised by progressive behavioural disturbance, dementia and chorea

AETIOLOGY

- Pathophysiology: **chr. 4p** codes for huntingtin protein. Triplet repeat **'CAG' expansions** within the huntingtin gene results in a toxic gain of function. This leads to accumulation of defective protein in neurons leading to GABA-ergic and cholinergic indirect striatal neuron atrophy → inhibitory pathways degenerate → hyperkinetic movements
- **Anticipation**: the number of trinucleotide repeat expansions ↑ in succeeding generations, leading to earlier age of onset and ↑severity

EPIDEMIOLOGY

- Worldwide prevalence: 8/100,000
- Average age of onset: 30–50 y/o (can be predicted by the number of **CAG repeats**)
- ♂ and ♀ are equally affected
- Rarer: juvenile onset (<20 y/o onset; 6% of all HD, the **Westphal variant**). These patients can additionally get Parkinsonism features presenting earlier

PRESENTATION

- Early disease: gradual onset with clumsiness, fidgetiness (typically the first feature) and irritability
- Late disease: progresses to:
  - **Dementia**:
    - Executive dysfunction: diminished ability to make decisions and multi-task
    - Patients typically lack insight into cognitive deficits
  - **Chorea**:
    - Involuntary, irregular, dance-like movements; mainly limbs and facial muscles:
      - ‡ Patients may be unaware of the movements and incorporate chorea into purposeful actions (known as parakinesia)
    - Chorea is worse with voluntary movement, disappears with sleep
    - Over time chorea becomes ↑widespread, progresses to dance-like movements or ballism (uncontrollable flailing of the extremities)
    - Late stage is replaced by dystonia and Parkinsonism features (such as bradykinesia, rigidity and postural instability), which are usually more disabling than the choreic phase
- Psychiatric symptoms: **depression**, impulsivity, personality change, psychosis:
  - May precede the onset of chorea by several years
- Weight loss and cachexia: these are commonly seen, despite appropriate caloric intake

INVESTIGATIONS

- Bloods: exclude other pathology, e.g. Wilson's disease, neuroacanthocytosis
- MRI brain: shows symmetrical atrophy of the striatum (caudate and putamen), hydrocephalus ex vacuo (**caudate nucleus** lies next to lateral ventricles so when they degenerate → ↑space in ventricles, i.e. **'box-car' ventricles**)
- Genetic analysis: diagnostic if there are >39 CAG repeats in the huntingtin gene

MANAGEMENT

- Purely symptomatic as there is no cure. An MDT approach is paramount
- Minimise chorea: dopamine-depleting drugs (**reserpine**, **tetrabenazine**) and benzodiazepines
- Psychological support: treat depression/psychosis (treat with atypical antidepressants to ↓risk of extrapyramidal side-effects)
- Genetic counselling: offer to family members

COMPLICATIONS

- 50% of offspring will carry the mutation in the huntingtin gene
- Psychological: ↑risk of depression and suicide (7%)

PROGNOSIS

- Life expectancy is approximately 20 years from the time of diagnosis
- Patients usually die from an intercurrent illness, e.g. respiratory tract infection

HYDROCEPHALUS

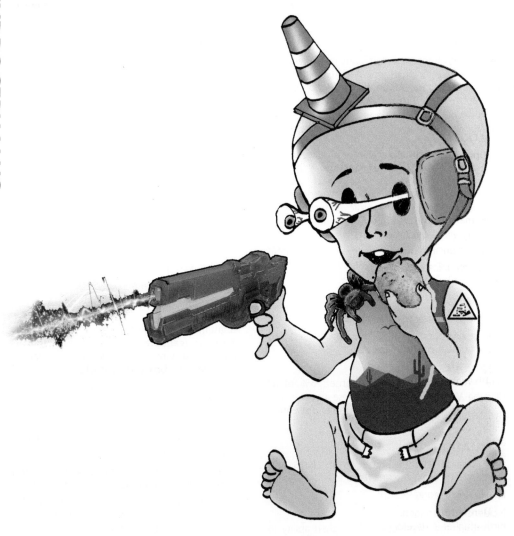

A baby has a large swollen head	**Hydrocephalus**
His eyes are popping out due to increased pressure	**Papilloedema**
He is holding and eating a potato tuber	**TB**
There is a tarantula on his shoulder	**SAH bleed** Arachnoid = tarantula
He is shooting a plasma gun in the right hand	**Toxoplasmosis** Toxo'plasm'osis = plasma gun
He is wearing horse 'blinders' preventing his ability to look laterally	**Horizontal diplopia (CN VI palsy)**
He is wearing a vest with a sunset design	**Sunset sign**
There is a tattoo on his shoulder of the safety acid symbol	**Acetazolamide** 'Acid'-azolamide
A tube leads from his head to his abdomen	**VP shunt**
There is a traffic cone on his head	**Coning**

HYDROCEPHALUS

DEFINITION

An abnormal accumulation of CSF within the ventricles of the brain, due to disturbance of CSF flow, absorption or (rarely) excessive production

AETIOLOGY

- Communicating (non-obstructive) hydrocephalus: ↓CSF absorption by arachnoid granulations → ↑ICP, **papilloedema** and eventual herniation:
  - Arachnoid scarring post meningitis (typically **TB**)
  - CNS tumours and **SAH bleed**
  - Normal pressure hydrocephalus
  - Rarely: CSF-secreting choroid plexus papilloma overproducing CSF
- Non-communicating (obstructive) hydrocephalus: structural blockage of CSF circulation within the ventricular system:
  - Lesions of the 3rd ventricle, 4th ventricle, cerebral aqueduct (e.g. stenosis of the aqueduct of Sylvius, colloid cyst of the 3rd ventricle)
  - Posterior fossa lesions (e.g. tumour, SAH bleed [↓ common as obstructive]) compressing the 4th ventricle
  - **Congenital toxoplasmosis**
- Hydrocephalus mimics: ex vacuo ventriculomegaly – apparent appearance of ↑CSF on imaging, but is actually due to central brain atrophy; seen in AD, advanced HIV, Pick's disease

EPIDEMIOLOGY

- Prevalence: 1%
- Incidence of congenital hydrocephalus: 1/1000 births (higher in developing countries)
- Bimodal age distribution; in the young: due to congenital malformations and tumours; in the elderly: due to tumours and strokes

PRESENTATION

- Communicating hydrocephalus:
  - Chronic cognitive decline. Hyper-reflexia may be seen, depending on the cause
  - Headaches may/may not be noted
- Non-communicating hydrocephalus:
  - Acute drop in conscious level
  - **Papilloedema**

- Diplopia: due **to VI nerve palsy ('false localising sign' of ↑ICP)**
  - VI cranial nerve has an abrupt bend before it enters the cavernous sinus, making it susceptible to compression with ↑ICP
- Neonates: enlargement of head circumference (crossing head growth centiles on the growth chart), **'sunset sign'**; impaired upward gaze
- Hydrocephalic attacks – abrupt LOC and collapse due to sudden ↑ICP:
  - Common in obstructive hydrocephalus, and is an ominous sign of worsening presentation
- Most often patients will present with a known history of hydrocephalus, where a treatment such as a VP shunt has failed leading to hydrocephalus recurrence

INVESTIGATIONS

- 1st line: CT head; detects hydrocephalus. CT may also detect the cause (e.g. tumour)
- CSF: sampled from ventricular drains or LP; indicated according to the underlying pathology (e.g. TB)
- LP: C/I in non-communicating hydrocephalus as it can lead to acute tonsillar herniation and death

MANAGEMENT

- Treat as an emergency
- Treat seizures. **Acetazolamide** ↓CSF production, isosorbide ↑CSF reabsorption (temporary measures)
- Urgent neurosurgery referral:
  - **VP shunting**: a catheter is placed leading from the lateral ventricles to a subcutaneous drain in the peritoneal cavity. These carry a risk of shunt infection, blockage or malfunction (some are electronic)
  - Advanced neurosurgery: endoscopic ventriculostomy/aqueductoplasty to bypass blockages

COMPLICATIONS

- Cerebral herniation, **coning** and death
- Hypopituitarism

PROGNOSIS

Obstructive hydrocephalus: this is often fatal if untreated (80%)

IDIOPATHIC INTRACRANIAL HYPERTENSION

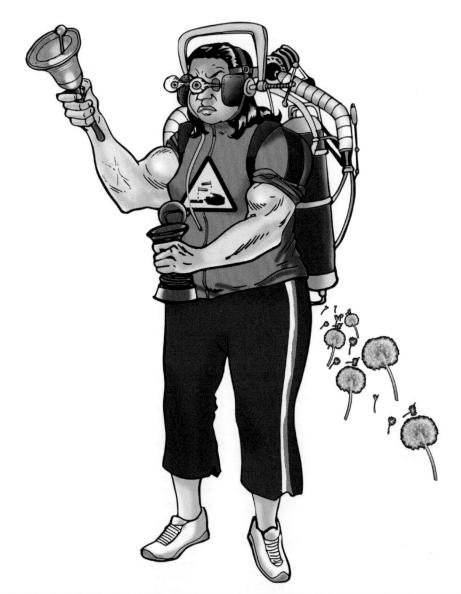

A woman with a large vice grip around her head	**Idiopathic intracranial hypertension, female** Vice grip causing increased tension around the cranium
She is obese and is holding a red tin	**Obesity, retinoids** Retinoids = red tin
Her biceps are huge	**Steroids (prednisolone)**
She is wearing a nitrous-powered jet pack	**Nitrofurantoin**
Her forehead is red due to headache, she is ringing a bell	**Headaches, tinnitus (pulsatile)**
Her eyes are popping out due to the increased pressure	**Papilloedema**
She is wearing horse 'blinders' either side of her face and is unable to look laterally	**Enlarged blind spot, horizontal diplopia**
Dandelions are coming out from the jet pack fumes	**Modified Dandy criteria**
She is wearing a safety acid logo on her top	**Acetazolamide**
A tube is running from her head to her abdomen	**VP shunt**

IDIOPATHIC INTRACRANIAL HYPERTENSION

DEFINITION
Raised ICP and papilloedema in the absence of a mass lesion or hydrocephalus

AETIOLOGY
- Pathophysiology: unknown; possible theories include excess vitamin A interfering with CSF resorption; alternatively, that **obesity** ↑intra-abdominal pressures → ↑cardiac filling pressures that impede cerebral venous return
- IIH associations:
  - Lateral venous sinus thrombosis
  - Habitus/diet: obesity, vitamin A toxicity **(retinoids)**
  - Endocrine: reproductive age, Addison's/ Cushing's disease, hyper/hypothyroidism
  - Haematological: iron deficiency anaemia, poly-cythaemia rubra vera
  - Drugs: COCP, **steroids** (administration or with-drawal), tetracyclines, **nitrofurantoin**
- Risk factors: similar to those for gallstones ('**fat, female**, fertile, forties')
- Also known as pseudotumour cerebri or benign intracranial hypertension (a misnomer as it is not a benign condition)

EPIDEMIOLOGY
- ♀:♂ = 3:1 to 8:1
- Peak incidence: 30–40 y/o
- Typically obese ♀ (90% of cases)

PRESENTATION
- **Headaches** (90%): usually the initial symptom:
  - Worst in the morning and at night, relieved by standing
  - Worsened by coughing, sneezing and positional changes as ↑ICP
- Visual features:
  - **Papilloedema** (usually bilateral and symmetri-cal), blurred vision and **enlarged blind spots**
  - **Horizontal diplopia from non-localising VI palsy**. This is because the CN VI is very thin, and has an abrupt angle of entry before it enters the cavernous sinus, making it susceptible to ↑ICP
  - Visual loss: usually gradual but can be abrupt (known as fulminant IIH; due to optic atrophy)
  - Poor colour vision and ↓visual acuity

- Retrobulbar pain (44%)
- Photopsia (~50%): presence of perceived flashes of light
- **Pulsatile tinnitus** (60%): pulse-synchronous whooshing sound, exacerbated with positional changes
- Dizziness
- Radicular pain, usually in the arms (uncommon symptom)

INVESTIGATIONS
- Diagnosis of exclusion: **modified Dandy criteria**
- Visual field charting: **enlarged blind spots** and peripheral field constriction is seen
- LP: opening pressure >20 cmH$_2$O is measured in the presence of normal CSF analysis
- CT/MRI brain: rules out hydrocephalus, mass or structural lesion
- MR venography: excludes venous sinus thrombosis

MANAGEMENT
- Acutely: **prednisolone**; relieves headaches and papilloedema (temporary measures prior to surgi-cal intervention)
- Conservative: weight loss and fluid/salt restriction. Stop offending medications. Ophthalmology follow-up
- Medical: **acetazolamide** (↓CSF production), consider furosemide as an adjunct or topiramate (relieves headache):
  - Indometacin: ↑cerebral vasoconstriction → ↓blood flow → ↓CSF pressure (not routinely used)
- Surgical: if resistant to the above: serial LPs or **VP shunt**:
  - If progressive impairment of visual acuity: optic nerve sheath fenestration
  - Bariatric surgery: currently undergoing clinical trials

COMPLICATIONS
Permanent blindness, seizures

PROGNOSIS
- Usually self-limiting
- Recurrence is common
- Permanent visual loss in 50%, and significant visual disability in 10%

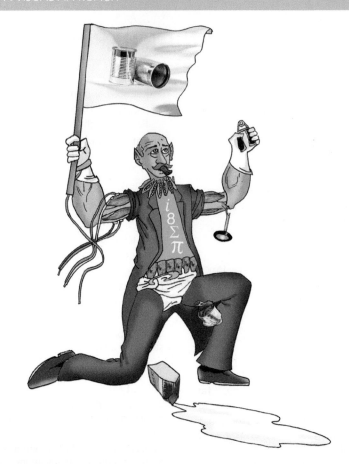

A butler is wearing an amber belt	**Lambert–Eaton myasthenic syndrome** L-amber-t belt; Lam'bert' similar to Butler
Around his neck there are peas 'queued' in a pod	**P/Q-type voltage calcium channels** Peas in a queue = P/Q
Near his right knee there is a carton of spilled milk	**↓Ca^{2+} influx** Milk = calcium; being poured out so less influx into the carton
The butler is in a lunge position, with a tin can squashed behind his left knee	**Small-cell lung cancer** Lunge = lung; tin can = cancer
He has larger forearms compared to his biceps	**Fatiguability of proximal muscles**
There is a broken tendon hammer lodged near the end of his left distal biceps tendons	**Depressed/absent deep tendon reflexes**
His tongue is dry and cracked	**Dry mouth**
He is compressing a hand grip in his left hand	**Lambert's sign**
He is holding up a flag with 2 tin cans	**Cancer is often discovered within the first 2 years of LEMS** 2 tin cans = 2 years in which cancer is diagnosed
Attached to his right arm there are electrical wires	**EMG**
He is wearing a diaper (nappy)	**3,4-DAP** DAP = diaper
He is wearing a T-shirt with a riddle on it involving 'π'	**Pyridostigmine** Pi-riddle = pyridostigmine. Answer: I ate some pie
He has ears like a goblin	**Igs** Immuno'globulin

LAMBERT–EATON MYASTHENIC SYNDROME

DEFINITION
Presynaptic autoantibodies occur against **P/Q-type voltage** calcium channels in the peripheral nervous system NMJ

AETIOLOGY
- Pathophysiology: antibodies directed against voltage-gated presynaptic calcium channels → ↓Ca^{2+} **influx** → ↓vesicles exocytose to release ACh to stimulate the postsynaptic membrane
- 60% are paraneoplastic; mainly **small-cell lung carcinoma** and to a lesser extent, breast and ovarian cancer:
  - Rapid progression suggests an associated cancer
  - Dysarthria, impotence and early involvement of distal muscles are also suggestive of rapid progression
- Can occur independently or alongside other autoimmune disorders, such as T1DM and thyroid disease

EPIDEMIOLOGY
- Prevalence: 0.4/100,000
- 20× less common than myasthenia gravis

PRESENTATION
- Weakness and **fatiguability of proximal muscles** along with **depressed/absent DTRs**:
  - Symptoms usually begin insidiously; many patients remain undiagnosed for months or years
  - Extra-ocular, respiratory and bulbar muscles are typically spared (unlike in myasthenia gravis)
  - Reflexes may return to normal after exercise (potentiation)
  - Limb girdle weakness (affects the lower limbs first); patients have difficulty climbing stairs and rising from a sitting position
- Autonomic symptoms (predominantly anti–cholinergic): micturition difficulties, impotence and **dry mouth**:
  - The parasympathetic system depends on ACh release to cause an effect on the target tissue This is depressed in LEMS
- Repeated muscle contractions lead to ↑muscle strength (postexercise enhancement), seen in 50% of patients. Roughly 5–10 s of rapid repetitive voluntary action leads to sufficient Ca^{2+} delivery to lead to a normal muscular contraction:

- **'Lambert's sign'**: improvement of power on repeated hand-grip
- Following prolonged effort, muscle strength will eventually↓
- Clinical manifestation frequently precedes cancer; in most cases a **cancer is discovered within the first 2 years of LEMS onset**. After 2 years, if no underlying malignancy is found it is likely to be due to an autoimmune aetiology

INVESTIGATIONS
- Bloods: exclude other causes of muscle disease (elevated CK may indicate myositis), TFTs (for thyrotoxic myopathy)
- Antibody assay: antibodies to VGCCs
- The most accurate test is **EMG**: repetitive nerve stimulation shows a characteristic incremental response (myasthenia gravis shows a decremental response)
- CT thorax: lung neoplasm; if nil found, a whole-body FDG-PET scan can be considered for occult malignancy

MANAGEMENT
- Manage underlying cause: e.g. **small-cell lung carcinoma**
- Symptomatic treatment: **3,4-DAP**, a K$^+$ channel blocker, causes hyperpolarisation → easier to reach the threshold to create an action potential) alongside **pyridostigmine** (AChE inhibitor)
- Immunosuppression: corticosteroids; in non-neoplastic cases, azathioprine, mycophenolate, etc
- Rescue therapy with plasma exchange and/or **Igs** may be beneficial; similar to myasthenia gravis
- Follow-up: repeat investigations/imaging for at least 5 years after diagnosis, as LEMS may precede the onset of detectable malignancy by several years

COMPLICATIONS
Paraneoplastic neuropathy

PROGNOSIS
- Dependent on the presence and nature of any underlying malignancy/the severity of associated autoimmune disease
- LEMS often leads to early detection of malignancy, therefore giving a better prognosis

MENINGITIS

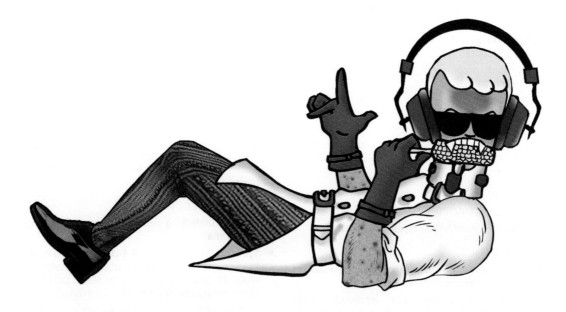

A man is wearing tights	**Meningitis** Man-in-tights
He has a red forehead and is wearing sunglasses to reduce the brightness	**Headaches, photophobia**
He is wearing a neck brace, making it difficult to move his neck	**Neck stiffness**
Has a non-blanching rash on his forearms	**Purpuric rash**
He is eating corn on the cob	**Kernig's sign** Kern = corn
His neck and hip are flexed	**Brudzinski's sign**
He is holding up his right hand, with fingers and thumb in 3 different axes	**Ceftriaxone** Cef-3 axes
His biceps are very muscular	**Steroids (dexamethasone)**
He is wearing industrial earmuffs	**Deafness**
He has sharp molar teeth like a vampire	**Rifampicin**
His head is quite large	**Hydrocephalus**

MENINGITIS

DEFINITION
Infection and/or inflammation of the leptomeninges (arachnoid and pia mater) surrounding the brain

AETIOLOGY
- Pathophysiology: haematogenous spread after invasion from a mucosal surface (nasopharynx) → organism enters the CSF via choroid plexus cells (as the BBB is vulnerable here). This excites an inflammatory response in the vascular pia; accumulation of exudate → obstructs CSF outflow (hydrocephalus), damages cranial nerves (CN VIII is commonly affected in children). Most damage occurs from the host response, not the infective organism
- Infection: (bacterial > viral > fungal):
  - 0–6 m/o (newborn): Group B *Streptococcus* > *E. coli* K1 > *Listeria*
  - 6 m–-6 y/o (children): *H. influenzae* type B > *S. pneumoniae*, *N. meningitidis* > Enteroviruses (Coxsackievirus)
  - 6–60 y/o: *N. meningitidis* (#1 in teens), *S. pneumoniae*, HSV and enteroviruses:
    - If there is suggestion of temporal lobe involvement (i.e. focal seizures), consider HSV as a likely cause
  - >60 y/o: *S. pneumoniae*, Gram –ve rods, *Listeria*. ↑risk with age-dependent immunity reduction
  - Immunocompromised: *S. pneumoniae*, *Cryptococcus neoformans*, MTB
- Endogenous: malignancy, autoimmune disease, subarachnoid haemorrhage
- Risk factors: sinusitis, inner ear infections, basal skull fractures, mastoiditis, immunocompromised

EPIDEMIOLOGY
- Affects all ages; young children and the elderly are predisposed
- Viral meningitis is most common, and is typically self-limiting. Bacterial tends to be ↑serious; ↓incidence of bacterial cases due to vaccination, especially *H. influenzae* meningitis

PRESENTATION
- Meningism: **headache, photophobia and neck stiffness**
- Septicaemia: fever, **purpuric rash (if meningococcal)**, hypotension (mortality doubles if septicaemia is present)
- ↑ICP: nerve palsies, N&V, seizures
- Signs of meningeal irritation:
  - **Kernig's sign**: resistance to knee extension when the hip is flexed to 90°
  - **Brudzinski's sign**: passive neck flexion causes involuntary hip and knee flexion
  - Jolt accentuation of headache manoeuvre: the patient rotates his head horizontally at 2–3 rotations/second. Exacerbation of headache is a +ve test. This is more sensitive than Brudzinski's and Kernig's sign

INVESTIGATIONS
- Blood cultures: 2 sets; do not delay antibiotics
- LP: CSF MC&S, Gram stain, glucose, viral serology, WBC, opening pressure (if suspect TB: AFB)
- If petechial rash + no clotting profile results (need to exclude DIC) → don't do an LP
- CT/MRI: exclude mass lesion, look for complications. If GCS ↓ → do CT prior to LP (to rule out an abscess)

MANAGEMENT
- Immediate: IV empirical antibiotics (treat immediately; don't wait for CT or LP results):
  - **Ceftriaxone** 2 g BD (or cefotaxime 2 g QDS) – always check your local hospital guidelines
  - Amoxicillin/benzylpenicillin can be given as initial blind therapy (especially if <3 m/o or >50 y/o)
  - Switch to the most appropriate antibiotic after blood /CSF culture results; continue for 14 days
- **Dexamethasone** IV ↓long-term complications (especially **deafness**). Avoid if HIV is suspected
- Notify public health and consult the ID consultant
- Chemoprophylaxis (e.g. **rifampicin**) for close contacts
- Prevention: meningococcal vaccine

COMPLICATIONS
- Hearing loss, especially with *S. pneumoniae* (the result of inflammatory damage to cochlear hair cells)
- Septicaemia, seizures, cerebral abscess/oedema, DIC
- **Hydrocephalus**, Waterhouse–Friderichsen syndrome

PROGNOSIS
- Viral meningitis is self-limiting (<10 days)
- Pneumococcal meningitis has a high mortality rate; however, if the patient recovers fully it has the lowest risk of long-term complications

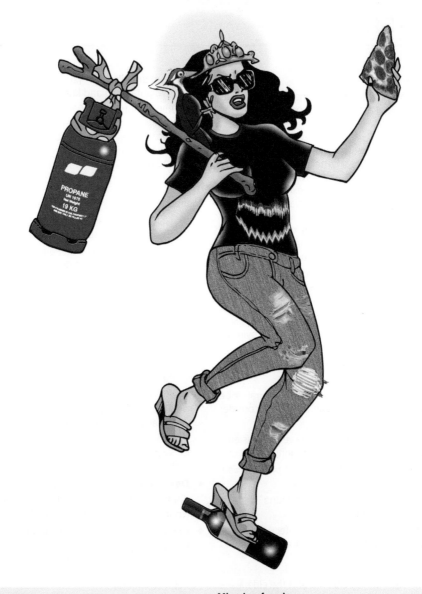

A migrant woman	**Migraine, female**
	She is migrating (a stick is over her shoulder)
She is wearing a 3-gemmed tiara	**Trigeminal nucleus**
	3-gem = 'trigem'inal nucleus
She is tripping over a bottle of red wine	**Triptans, red wine**
	Tripping = triptans
A woodpecker is pecking the right side of her head	**Unilateral throbbing headache**
There is an aura around her head	**Aura**
She is wearing a T-shirt with a zigzag design	**Fortification spectra/scintillating scotoma**
She is wearing sunglasses to shield her eyes from lights	**Photophobia**
She is carrying a propane gas tank over her shoulder	**Propanolol**
	Propane = propanolol
She is holding a slice of pizza in her left hand	**Pizotifen**
	Pizza = 'pizo'tifen

MIGRAINE

DEFINITION

An episodic headache syndrome, often associated with N&V and visual disturbance. The name is derived from the greek 'hemicrania', as it tends to affect one-half of the head

AETIOLOGY

- Pathophysiology: cortical spreading depression theory – a wave of hyperexcitability through the cortex → constricts blood vessels → ischaemia → aura. Also activates and sensitises the **trigeminal nucleus**, leading to vasoactive peptides (CGRP, substance P) causing vasodilation, which further compresses on the nucleus to cause pain
- Triggers: certain foods (e.g. **red wine**, cheese, processed meats, chocolate), stress, menstruation, bright lights, caffeine withdrawal, sleep excess/deprivation and COCP (C/I with complicated migraine due to stroke risk)

EPIDEMIOLOGY

- 18% in ♀, 6% in ♂ (3:1); frequency ↓ with age, especially at the menopause
- Familial predisposition: 50% have an affected family member

PRESENTATION

- Classical migraine: triad of:
  - Headache: disabling, paroxysmal **unilateral throbbing headache**:
    - Lasts 4–72 hours, bilateral in 30–40%
  - Aura (focal neurological deficit): flashing lights, **fortification spectra/scintillating scotoma** or unusual smells:
    - Occurs 15–60 min prior to headache
  - N&V, **photophobia** and/or phonophobia
- Common migraine: same as classical migraine except no aura (diad)
- Complicated migraine: with severe/persistent sensorimotor deficits:
  - Basilar-type migraine: occipital headache with diplopia, vertigo, ataxia and altered level of consciousness
  - Hemiplegic/hemisensory migraine: rare (can be familial or sporadic), follows attack. Mimics stroke

- Ophthalmoplegic migraine
- Acephalgic migraine ('silent migraine'): aura without headache. May experience N&V or photophobia/phonophobia
- Menstrual migraine: migraine at menstruation onset, usually 2 days prior to 3 days after menstruation
- When attacks occur for ≥15 days/month, it is called chronic migraine

INVESTIGATIONS

- Diagnosis is based on the history
- Investigations are used to exclude other diagnoses:
  - CT/MRI brain, if secondary headache disorders are suspected

MANAGEMENT

- Acute migraine:
  - Best initial management: oral sumatriptan and oral NSAID; most cost and clinically effective:
    - Relieve pain (simple analgesics), antiemetic if vomiting
    - Abortive treatment; **triptans**: these vasoconstrict to reduce the pain; hence why triptans are C/I for arterial disease (MI, stroke)
- Long-term management:
  - Avoid known triggers, stress reduction
  - If >2/mo: indication for prophylactic medication; **propranolol**, CCB, **pizotifen** (5-HT$_2$ antagonist), topiramate (AED)
  - Riboflavin OD may be effective in reducing migraine frequency and intensity

COMPLICATIONS

- Disruption of daily activities
- Chronic use of analgesics can progress to analgesia-overuse headache

PROGNOSIS

Long-term; majority of causes are well managed by preventative measures

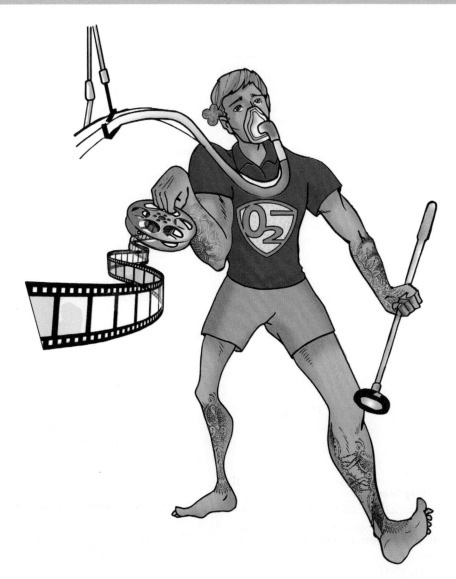

A man with lots of Mehndi tattoos across his body	**Motor neuron disease** 'Mehndi' sounded out similar to MND
He is wearing a T-shirt with an 'O$_2$·' logo	**SOD mutation** 'O$_2$·' is a symbol for free radical superoxide
He has a muscle-wasted left upper limb and right lower limb	**LMN lesion signs (e.g. muscle wasting), asymmetrical involvement**
He has a muscular right upper limb and left lower limb	**UMN lesion signs; asymmetrical involvement** Follows a pyramidal pattern, i.e. the right upper limb is flexed
A tendon hammer is striking his left knee	**Hyper-reflexia; UMN sign**
His left lower foot is showing a +ve Babinski sign	**Babinski sign +ve**
He has a 4-leaf clover over his ear	**Baclofen** Ba'clofen' sounds out similar to clover
He is holding a movie reel in his right hand	**Riluzole** Movie 'reel'-uzole
He is wearing a non-invasive ventilation mask	**Respiratory failure**

MOTOR NEURON DISEASE

DEFINITION

A progressive, neurodegenerative disorder of various subtypes, with differing involvement of cortical, brainstem and spinal motor neurons (purely motor)

AETIOLOGY

- Pathophysiology: 20 genes are known to cause MND; the most common mutations are in *SOD1*, *C9orf72*, *TARDBP* and *FUS* genes. **SOD1 gene mutation** causes a toxic gain of function → cannot convert superoxide (O_2^-) free radical into non-toxic products → damage to motor neurons
- Unknown; sporadic in 95% of cases; familial in 5–10% of cases
- Progressive motor neuron loss with astrocytic gliosis (replaces lost neurons)

EPIDEMIOLOGY

- Incidence: 2/100,000 annually (rare)
- Mean onset: 55 y/o
- ♂:♀ = 1.6:1

PRESENTATION

- Amyotrophy (muscle wasting) lateral (corticospinal tracts) sclerosis (scarring); ALS is the most common subtype (75%). In most instances MND and ALS are used interchangeably:
  - **Mixture of UMN and LMN signs; often asymmetrical involvement of the limbs**
  - Can be present in the same muscle:
    - UMN features: spastic or pyramidal pattern of weakness, **brisk reflexes, +ve Babinski sign**
    - LMN features: **muscle wasting**, fasciculations, flaccid weakness
- Progressive muscular atrophy: isolated LMN signs (e.g. flail arm/foot). Good prognosis
- Primary lateral sclerosis: isolated UMN signs; degeneration of corticospinal tracts; slower disease progression
- PSP: bulbar signs; wasted tongue (LMN), brisk jaw jerk (UMN). Poor prognosis

- There is no sensory loss and sphincters are spared; if these are present consider other causes

INVESTIGATIONS

- Bloods: show ↑CK (due to muscle breakdown)
- EMG: demonstrates widespread denervation (nerve conduction studies are often normal)
- Muscle biopsy: shows neurogenic atrophy
- MRI of the brain and spinal cord: exclude structural pathology, cord/root compression
- Spirometry: measures FVC to assess the level of respiratory compromise

MANAGEMENT

- MDT approach: Neuromuscular neurologist, MND nurses, psychological support, PT, OT, SALT
- Symptomatic: spasticity (**baclofen**), salivation (anticholinergics)
- **Riluzole** (inhibits voltage-gated Na⁺ channels and glutamate transmission); modest survival ↑:
  - Prescribed early in disease (does not reverse damage); requires regular LFT monitoring
  - Prolongs life by ~3 months but does not improve function or quality of life and is costly
- Non-invasive ventilation: usually BiPAP at night: studies show a survival benefit of ~7 months
- Later stages: consider PEG feed. Palliative care in terminal cases

COMPLICATIONS

- Depression, may be associated with frontotemporal dysfunction/dementia, weight loss and malnutrition (2° to dysphagia)
- Common cause of death: **respiratory failure** due to respiratory muscle weakness

PROGNOSIS

At present MND is an incurable, progressive disease (mean survival = 3 years)

MULTIPLE SCLEROSIS

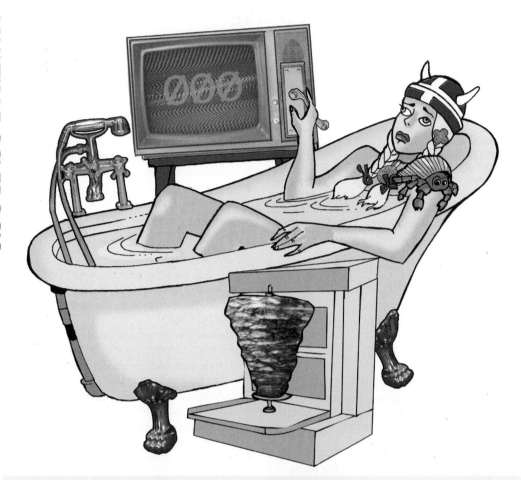

A TV has multiple 'zeros' on the screen	**Multiple sclerosis** Sclero sounds like zero
A woman is wearing a helmet with devil horns	**Devic's disease**
She is a young, Caucasian blonde woman in a bathtub	**Young, Caucasian female** (the typical MS patient)
Her eyes are in a characteristic position	**Internuclear ophthalmoplegia**
Her hat has the Danish flag on it	**DANISH cerebellar signs**
She has had a urinary accident in the bath, seen by the yellow water discolouration	**Urinary urgency/hesistancy**
She has her clothes off, taking a hot bath	**Uhthoff's phenomenon** Hot bath, clothes off = Uhtoff
On her left shoulder there is a hermit crab	**Lhermitte's sign**
She has a sad face	**Depression**
By the bathtub there is a doner kebab on a vertical rotisserie	**Doner = McDonald's criteria**
She is turning a door handle in an attempt to make the TV work	**Dawson's fingers** 'Daw'son = door
The TV screen is showing interference	**Interferon-β**
She is wearing a talisman around her neck	**Natalizumab** Talisman = na'talizum'ab
She has a clover leaf over her ear	**Baclofen**

MULTIPLE SCLEROSIS

DEFINITION
A chronic, autoimmune destruction of CNS myelin and oligodendrocytes (white matter demyelination)

AETIOLOGY
- Pathophysiology: unknown; possibly asymptomatic infection → Ab production → autoimmune response 2° to molecular mimicry between antigens on infective organism and antigens on oligodendrocytes and CNS myelin. Normally macrophages cannot easily cross the BBB, but in MS they express adhesion proteins (glycoprotein $\alpha4$ $\beta1$) allowing them to cross the endothelium → inflammatory damage and plaque formation
- Risk factors: HLA-DR2, EBV exposure and ↓vitamin D levels have been implicated
- MS clinical progression types:
  - Relapsing-remitting: unpredictable attacks +/- permanent deficits, followed by periods of remission (80%):
    - Unpredictable attacks; on average occur every 1.5 years (duration of 6–8 weeks)
  - 2° Progressive: initial relapsing-remitting that progresses without periods of remission
  - 1° Progressive: steady ↑ in disability without attacks (10–20%)
  - Progressive relapsing: steady decline from onset with super imposed attacks (<10%)
- MS variants:
  - **Devic's disease** (neuromyelitis optica): severe optic nerve and spinal cord involvement
  - Tumefactive MS: solitary lesion >2 cm. Can mimic neoplasms on MRI
  - Fulminant MS: rapidly progressive and fatal MS associated with severe axonal damage and inflammation
  - ADEM: monophasic demyelinating disease, usually post viral infection, that leads to sudden multi-focal neurological deficits with rapid deterioration

EPIDEMIOLOGY
- Prevalence: 1/1000
- Onset is 20–40 y/o
- Highest risk is in **Caucasians**
- Common in **young ♀**
- Incidence ↑ as move further away from the equator

PRESENTATION
- Multiple neurological complaints separated in time and space; not explained by a single lesion
- Eye signs: optic neuritis (commonest), RAPD, central scotoma

- **Internuclear opthalmoplegia**: bilateral strongly suggests MS
- Motor: UMN signs; spastic paresis, brisk reflexes
- Sensory: paraesthesia; ↓vibration sensation
- Cerebellar: **DANISH signs**:
  - **D**ysdiadochokinesia, **A**taxia, **N**ystagmus, **I**ntention tremor, **S**lurred speech and **H**ypotonia
- Autonomic: **urinary urgency/hesistancy**, bowel dysfunction
- **Uhthoff's phenomenon**: ↑body temperatures worsens symptoms, such as exercising or taking a hot bath
- **Lhermitte's sign**: shooting electric shock-like pain down the arms and legs on cervical flexion due to cervical cord plaques
- Psychological: depression, cognitive impairment

INVESTIGATIONS
- Clinical diagnosis; two or more CNS lesions separated in time and space (**McDonald's criteria**)
- Best initial/most accurate test: MRI brain; shows multiple lesions; active lesions enhance with gadolinium:
  - Often shows periventricular plaques radiating from the corpus callosum = **Dawson's fingers**
- If MRI is non-diagnostic: LP; oligoclonal IgG bands; visual evoked potentials show ↓central conduction velocity

MANAGEMENT
- Acute exacerbation: IV high-dose methylprednisolone; if poor response and severe deficit, consider plasma exchange
- MDT approach: specialist nurses, PT, pain team and psychologists
- 1st line treatment: **interferon-β** (inhibits T cell activation; apoptosis of autoreactive T cells):
  - If poor response: **natalizumab** (a monoclonal antibody [anti-α4 antigen] that inhibits T cell movement into the CNS)
  - Other disease-modifying agents are now available, e.g. dimethyl fumarate
- Symptomatic: spasticity: **baclofen**; fatigue: modafinil; depression: consider antidepressants

COMPLICATIONS
- Progression of disability, cognitive impairment
- **Natalizumab** has 1/1000 risk of causing progressive multifocal leukoencephalopathy

PROGNOSIS
Best with a relapsing and remitting history; MS is likely to progress to 2° progressive MS in 80% of cases within 20 years

MYASTHENIA GRAVIS

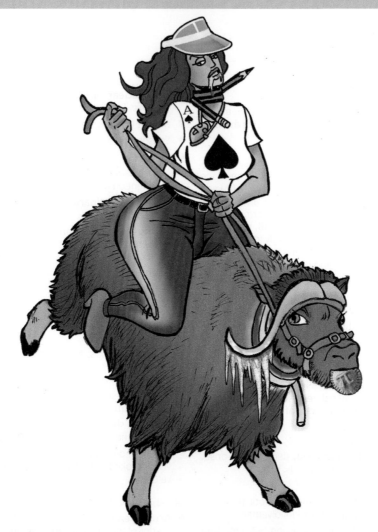

A woman is wearing a visor hat	**Myasthenia gravis** Gra'vis' = visor
She has large thighs	**Thymus association** 'Thigh'-mus
There is a pencil around her neck	**Penicillamine**
She is a young female	**Young female**
Her eyelids are both drooping and there is a squint; her head is tilted upwards	**Ptosis and diplopia; compensatory head tilt**
She is snarling and drooling; her neck is constricted making it difficult to swallow	**Myasthenic snarl, dysphagia, drooling**
She is wearing an Ace T-shirt and is riding a musk ox	**ACh receptor antibodies, anti-MuSK antibodies** Ace =' ace'tylcholine receptor
She is holding tightly onto the reins	**Tensilon test** Creating tension with the reins
The musk ox's horns are frozen with icicles	**Ice pack test**
There is an oxygen mask around the woman's neck	**Respiratory compromise**
There is a neon ring around the musk ox's neck. The musk ox is eating a 'π' pie	**Neostigmine, pyridostigmine** 'Neon'-stigmine; 'π'-ridostigmine

MYASTHENIA GRAVIS

DEFINITION
An autoimmune disorder characterised by weakness and fatiguability of skeletal muscles due to dysfunction of the NMJ

AETIOLOGY
- Pathophysiology: B and T cell-mediated IgG autoantibodies attack the postsynaptic ACh receptors at the NMJ → early saturation of the NMJ and inadequate muscle activation with ↑nerve stimulation
- Mainly idiopathic, linked with other autoimmune conditions
- **Thymus association**; 75% have thymic hyperplasia, 10% have thymoma
- Rarely, can be induced/aggravated by drug treatment: **penicillamine** (well documented), β-blockers, CCB, gentamicin and lithium

EPIDEMIOLOGY
- Prevalence: 1/5000
- Bimodal distribution: **young ♀** and old ♂

PRESENTATION
- Muscle weakness; worsens as the day progresses (fatiguability) and improves with rest, e.g. in the morning/after a nap (rest replenishes ACh)
- Affected muscle groups:
  - Ocular: **ptosis** and **diplopia (may tilt head upwards to compensate)**
  - Bulbar: facial weakness (**myasthenic snarl** on attempting to smile), dysarthria, **dysphagia** and **drooling**
  - Proximal muscles: shoulder and thighs
  - Axial muscles: neck and trunk, including respiratory muscles
- Usually tone, reflexes and sensation are normal

INVESTIGATIONS
- Fatiguability tests (muscle weakness due to fatiguability will improve with rest or ice):
  - Eyes: the patient is asked to sustain an upgaze for 30 seconds → ptosis or diplopia
    - Best initial test: **ice pack test**; crushed ice is placed in a latex glove and applied to the eye for 3 minutes; improves ptosis (sensitivity and specificity of >90%)
  - Speech (bulbar): the patient is asked to count to 50 → dysarthria
  - Arms (proximal muscles): the patient is asked to repeatedly shoulder abduct (20–30×); strength is assessed before and after
- Edrophonium *aka* **Tensilon test**: short-acting AChE inhibitor. If the patient has myasthenia gravis, dramatic symptomatic improvement for several minutes will occur. AChE inhibitor ↑ risk of bradycardia, hence may need to administer atropine
- **ACh receptor antibodies** +ve (if –ve, check for **anti-MuSK** antibodies)
- Most accurate test: single-fibre EMG; shows a decremental response with repeating testing, ↑'jitter' at the NMJ
- Spirometry: serial FVCs to check for **respiratory compromise**:
  - If unable to access spirometry, a 'single-breath test' can be performed as a bedside test; the patient is asked to take a single deep breath in and then count from 1 to 50 in that single breath:
    - If they are able to count to 40–50, there is no need to worry. Counting to <15 indicates a dangerously low FVC
- CT thorax: evaluates for thymoma. Note that contrast can exacerbate myasthenia gravis

MANAGEMENT
- Symptomatic relief: **pyridostigmine** (most commonly used) and **neostigmine** – both are long-acting AChE inhibitors
- Immunosuppression: steroids (mainstay of treatment) and other immunosuppressants
- Thymectomy: can be curative

COMPLICATIONS
- Myasthenic crisis: respiratory compromise and aspiration; treat with IVIG/plasmapheresis
- Cholinergic crisis: NMJ overstimulation 2° to AChE inhibitors; flaccid paralysis
- Neonatal myasthenia crisis: autoantibodies cross the placenta → transient fatiguability symptoms in the baby

PROGNOSIS
- With treatment, life expectancy is normal
- There is a 30% spontaneous remission

MYOTONIC DYSTROPHY

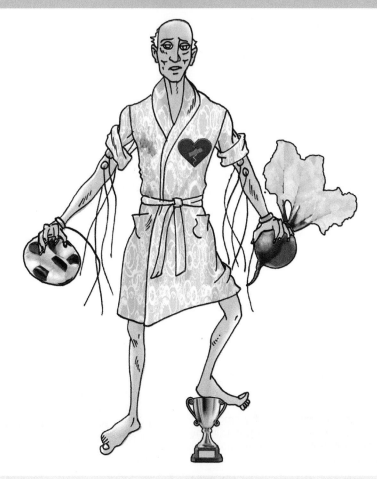

A man is leaning on a trophy	**Myotonic dystrophy** Dys'trophy'
He has cottage cheese dripping from his clothes	**CTG triplet repeat** CoTtaGe = CTG repeat
He has cute dimples	***DMPK* gene** DiMPles = DMPK
In his left hand, his is holding a beetroot; one of his fingers looks made out of metal	**Insulin resistance (diabetes mellitus), ZNF9** Dia'beet'es, ZNF9 = zinc (metal) finger
His face looks wasted and expressionless; he has bilateral droopy eyelids	**Facial muscle weakness, bilateral ptosis, expressionless face**
He is balding from the front	**Frontal balding**
His hands look like claws because he cannot relax his grip	**Inability to release grip**
He has difficulty lifting his arms	**Distal weakness**
Both his eyes are cloudy	**Subcapsular cataracts**
His heart is broken with a plaster on it	**Cardiac conduction defect**
In his right hand he is holding a deflated football	**Hypogonadism (testicular atrophy)** Foot'ball' to symbolise gonads
He has wires dangling from both his arms	**EMG**
His big toe bilaterally is very large	**Phenytoin** Toin = toe

MYOTONIC DYSTROPHY

DEFINITION

An autosomal dominant triplet repeat (CTG) expansion myopathy, characterised by slowly progressive muscle wasting, weakness and myotonia (abnormally prolonged muscle contraction)

AETIOLOGY

- Pathophysiology: triplet repeat expansion dysregulates gene transcription/translation of myocyte regulatory proteins
- *Aka* Dystrophia myotonica (DM); there are two main types:
  - DM1: **CTG triplet repeat expansion** in **DMPK gene** on chr. 19:
    - Exhibits anticipation: earlier onset/↑severity in offspring as result of increasing triplet repeat expansions within the gene
    - Distal weakness is prominent
  - DM2: CTG triplet repeat expansion in **ZNF9 gene** on chr. 3:
    - Proximal weakness is prominent
    - Rarer; ↓severe than DM1

EPIDEMIOLOGY

- Most common adult inherited myopathy
- Annual incidence: 1/8000
- Onset: DM1 20–50 y/o (DM2 later) but variable, depending on the number of triplet repeats

PRESENTATION

- Appearance:
  - Myopathic facies: **facial muscle wasting** and **weakness** and **bilateral ptosis** → **expressionless face**:
    - Wasting of frontalis, temporalis and sternocleidomastoid muscles
  - **Frontal balding** (in both sexes)
- Musculoskeletal:
  - Myotonia (delayed muscle relaxation after contraction): a hallmark of this condition:
    - Can be elicited by a hand-shake followed by an **inability to release the grip**
    - Percussion myotonia: striking the thenar eminence → slow thumb flexion
  - **Distal weakness in DM1**: distal weaker than proximal (in contrast to other myopathies) with arreflexia:
    - Specifically finger/wrist extensors, ankle dorsiflexors; may see a high stepping gait
- Cognitive: mild mental impairment
- Ocular: **subcapsular cataracts**, retinal degeneration
- Cardiac: 90% have **conduction defects** (heart block, atrial arrhythmia), cardiomyopathy
- Respiratory: hypoventilation 2° to muscle weakness
- Endocrinopathy: **hypogonadism (testicular atrophy), insulin resistance**
- Gastrointestinal: oesophageal dysfunction, dysphagia, pseudo-obstruction

INVESTIGATIONS

- Bloods: CK (may be ↑)
- ECG (annual): screens for cardiac conduction defects
- Echo: if there are indications of myocardial dysfunction
- FVC: checks for respiratory compromise
- **EMG**: shows 'dive-bomber' potentials long runs with declining frequency and amplitude
- Gene analysis: for CTG triplet repeat expansion

MANAGEMENT

- MDT approach is best (PT/OT/SALT). Weakness is the major problem as there is no treatment
- Low-intensity exercise training programme (if no severe cardiac defects)
- Severe myotonia: adults → **phenytoin**, children → mexiletine (1b antiarrhythmic)
- Genetic counselling

COMPLICATIONS

- Cardiorespiratory complications: cause of death in >50%
- Neurological, endocrine and cardiac complications as mentioned above
- ↑Risk of complications (cardiac/respiratory) with general anaesthesia

PROGNOSIS

Most patients do not survive beyond 50 y/o

NEUROFIBROMATOSIS

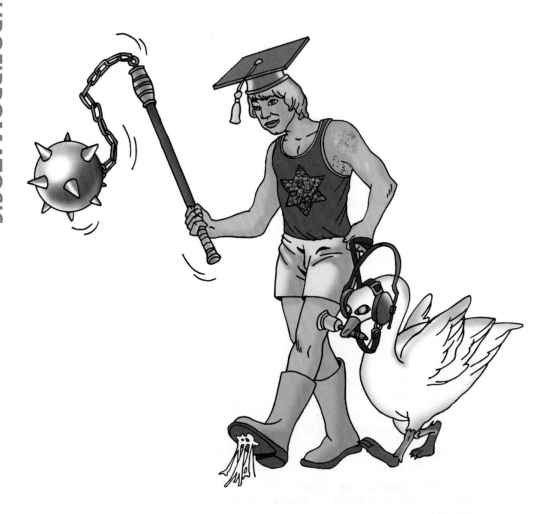

A man is swinging a wrecking ball	**Von Recklinghausen's disease (NF1)** Wrecking = Reckling
He is wearing a vest with a 6-pointed star with coffee bean design	**Café-au-lait spots ≥6**
He has freckling underneath his armpits	**Freckling**
Neurofibromas can be seen on his left shoulder	**Neurofibromas ≥2**
He has stepped in some glue, which is stuck to his foot	**Optic nerve glioma** Glue = glioma
A swan is attached to the man by a leash	**Lisch nodules**
The man has a bent back; he can't stand up straight	**Scoliosis**
He is wearing a graduation degree hat	**1st degree relatives**
The swan is wearing industrial earmuffs	**Schwannoma, hearing loss**
Its eyes have cataracts; it is holding a bell in its beak	**Juvenile cataracts, tinnitus**

NEUROFIBROMATOSIS

DEFINITION
A neurocutaneous genetic disorder arising from mutated tumour suppressor (NF) genes

AETIOLOGY
- Pathophysiology:
  - NF1: *NF1* gene (on chr. 17) encodes neurofibromin (a GTPase activator). *NF1* mutation → loss of GTPase activity → ↑p21-ras proto-oncogene activity
  - NF2: *NF2* gene (on chr. 22) encodes merlin (*aka* schwannomin; a scaffolding protein). *NF2* mutation → abnormal cell growth
- Autosomal dominant (50%), or *de novo* (50%) mutations in tumour suppressor genes *NF1* or *NF2*
- 100% penetrant; variable expression

EPIDEMIOLOGY
- NF1 incidence: 1/3000
- NF2 incidence: 1/40,000

PRESENTATION
- NF1; *aka* **von Recklinghausen's disease**: largely skin lesions
- NF1 diagnostic criteria: need 2/7. Most patients are diagnosed after puberty; they may not have all the features before puberty:
  - 1 **Café-au-lait spots** ≥6 (each must be ≥5 mm in children, ≥15 mm in adults)
  - 2 **Freckling**: axillary or inguinal
  - 3 **Neurofibromas** ≥2: either dermal (rarely malignant) or plexiform (↑malignant potential)
  - 4 **Optic nerve glioma**: causes asymmetrical visual field defects, precocious puberty (due to pituitary chiasm compression)
  - 5 **Lisch nodules** ≥2: *aka* iris hamartomas; seen best on slit lamp examination
  - 6 **Skeletal deformities**; e.g. **spinal scoliosis**, sphenoid dysplasia
  - 7 **1st degree relative** with NF1
- NF2: largely CNS lesions
- NF2 diagnostic criteria: need 1/3:
  - 1 **Bilateral acoustic neuroma**; *aka* **vestibular schwannoma** (slow-growing tumour of CN VIII):
    - **Bilateral sensorineural hearing loss, tinnitus,** vertigo. Acoustic neuroma = misnomer, as the tumour typically arises from the vestibular, not cochlear (acoustic), portion of CN VIII:

- ‡ Begins in the internal auditory meatus. Over time it expands into the cerebellopontine angle → compressing the cerebellum and brainstem → CN V–VII compression. Ataxia may occur (due to cerebellar compression)
- ‡ Absent corneal reflex (CN V_1) + facial palsy (CN VII) are important late signs
  - 2 Unilateral CN VIII mass + 1st degree relative with NF2:
  - 3 ≥2 of following below + 1st degree relative with NF2:
    - Meningioma, glioma, **schwannoma, juvenile cataracts** (usually the first sign to occur)

INVESTIGATIONS
- Ophthalmology and audiometry assessment
- MRI internal auditory canal/cerebellopontine angle: shows **schwannomas**
- Skull X-ray: shows sphenoid dysplasia
- Genetic testing: can be difficult as the *NF1* gene is very long

MANAGEMENT
- There is no cure; symptomatic treatment only. The mainstay is education and surveillance for complications
- NF1: regular height/weight and pubertal development assessment. Monitor skin lesions and visual symptoms
- NF2: Regular hearing assessments. MRI follow-up of CNS lesions
- Surgery: decompress acoustic neuromas (also consider stereotactic radiosurgery), remove disfiguring tumours, treat skeletal abnormalities
- Genetic counselling prior to conception: 50% risk of passing to offspring

COMPLICATIONS
- NF1: learning difficulties, congenital heart disease (pulmonary stenosis), plexiform neurofibroma malignancy
- NF2: ↑risk of brain tumours

PROGNOSIS
- NF1: shortened life expectancy
- NF2: worse prognosis than NF1
- If no disease is found at 20 y/o → low risk of NF. No disease at 30 y/o: almost guarantees that the mutated gene has not been inherited

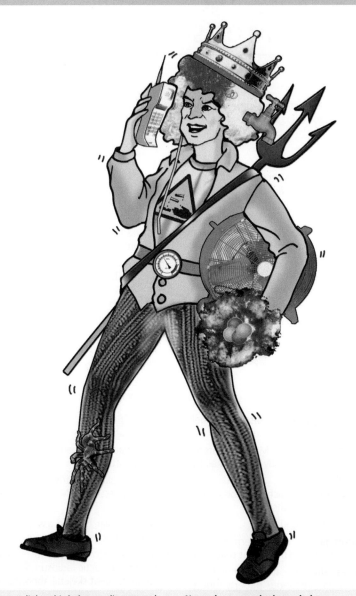

A man with a pressure dial on his belt recording normal range	**Normal pressure hydrocephalus**
He is holding a mobile phone	**Communicating (hydrocephalus)**
He is holding a large ventilator fan under his arm	**Ventricular enlargement**
He is wearing a crown that is too big for his head	**Corona radiata (dilated)**
He has wet himself, is wobbling and has wacky-coloured, curly hair	**Wet, wobbly and wacky**
There is a tarantula crawling up his tights	**Subarachnoid (haemorrhage), meningitis**
There is a demon trident on his back	**Dementia**
His feet are far apart	**Wide stance**
There is an old-style tap attached to his hair	**Lumbar tap test**
There is a fusion reaction occurring in his left hand	**Lumbar infusion test**
He is wearing a T-shirt with a safety acid symbol	**Acetazolamide**
A tube leads from his head to his abdomen	**VP shunt**

NORMAL PRESSURE HYDROCEPHALUS

DEFINITION

A potentially reversible form of dementia, due to impaired CSF outflow leading to chronic ventricular enlargement

AETIOLOGY

- Pathophysiology: **communicating hydrocephalus**; ↓absorption of CSF through arachnoid granulations → **expansion of ventricles** → distortion of long white matter tracts (**corona radiata**, anterior commissure)
- Leads to the clinical triad of urinary incontinence, ataxia and cognitive dysfunction (sometimes reversible), '**wet, wobbly and wacky**'
- Causes: 50% are idiopathic; 50% due to: **SAH, meningitis**, trauma, radiation-induced
- CSF pressure is ↑ (150–200 mmH$_2$O); however, this is within the normal CSF pressure range, hence 'normal pressure' hydrocephalus

EPIDEMIOLOGY

- Prevalence: 0.5% in >65 y/o
- Accounts for 6% of **dementias**

PRESENTATION

- The classical triad (not pathognomonic). Gradually progressive:
  - Apraxic gait; usually the first presentation. Most responsive to treatment:
    - **Wide stance**, short steps – classically described as 'magnetic' or 'feet glued to the floor', as the forefoot is not completely dorsally extended
    - Due to distortion of the sacral motor fibres that innervate the legs
  - Urinary incontinence:
    - Spastic hyper-reflexic bladder; ↑urgency
    - In combination with frontal lobe impairment; 'frontal lobe incontinence' – the patient becomes indifferent to urinary incontinence symptoms

- **Dementia**; usually the last presentation. Most refractory to treatment:
  - Distortion of the periventricular limbic system
  - Dementia progresses less rapidly compared to AD
- Headaches and other signs of ↑ICP (e.g. papilloedema) typically do not appear, although continuous ICP monitoring may reveal spikes of elevated pressure (>200 mmH$_2$O)

INVESTIGATIONS

- Largely a clinical diagnosis
- Best initial test: CT/MRI head; shows **ventricular enlargement** out of proportion to sulcal atrophy; rules out other causes; mass lesions
- **Lumbar tap test**/Miller Fisher test: assessment of the clinical picture alongside continuous lumbar CSF drainage. If symptoms improve, it is used as a predictor of +ve surgical shunting outcome
- **Lumbar infusion test**: measures CSF absorptive capacity with a fluid challenge; an abnormal sustained rise in CSF suggests normal pressure hydrocephalus. It has a higher sensitivity and specificity compared to the lumbar tap test

MANAGEMENT

- Medical treatment: **acetazolamide** and repeated LP (in patients unable to undergo surgery)
- Definitive management: **VP shunt** (choroid plexectomy in some cases)

COMPLICATIONS

Following shunt surgery: shunt occlusion, CSF hypotensive headaches, haemorrhage and seizures

PROGNOSIS

- Following shunt surgery: 1/5th of patients show marked improvement in symptoms
- Long-term survival: 39% after 5 years

OSMOTIC DEMYELINATION SYNDROME

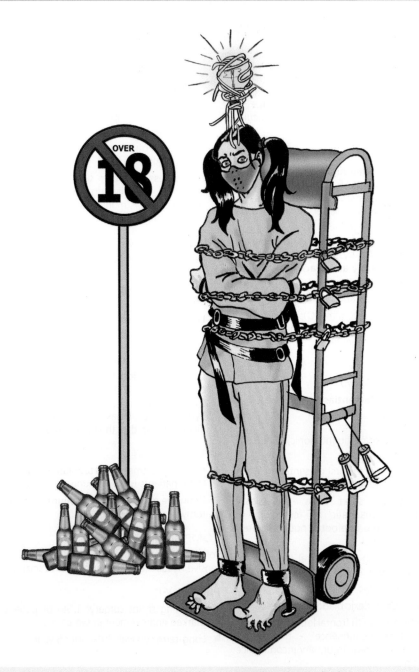

A woman with hair ponytails is wearing a straight-jacket	**Central pontine myelinolysis** Pontine = ponytails
Attached to a trolley there are empty salt shakers	**Hyponatraemia**
There are multiple alcoholic beer bottles piled up	**Alcoholism**
She cannot move her arms and legs, and her toes are fanned out	**Spastic quadriparesis**
She is having a light bulb moment, where the bulb has udon noodles wrapped around it	**Pseudobulbar palsy** loosely sounds like udo(n) and nood-le, wrapped around a bulb-ar
She is chained up with chains and locks	**Locked-in syndrome**
A sign to her right says 'no over 18s'	**No more than 18 mmol/l in 1st 48 h**

OSMOTIC DEMYELINATION SYNDROME

DEFINITION

A symmetrical, non-inflammatory acute demyelination of the pons (anterior brainstem) typically with rapid correction of hyponatraemia. It has replaced the term central pontine myelinolysis, as this pathology can also occur outside of the pons

AETIOLOGY

- Pathophysiology:
  - **Hyponatraemia** ($\downarrow$Na$^+$) → $\downarrow$serum osmolality → water flows across BBB → $\uparrow$brain water content
  - The brain has adaptive mechanisms to prevent severe cerebral oedema due to chronic hyponatraemia that develops over >2–3 days:
    - $\uparrow$ICP forces interstitial Na$^+$ and water into CSF → $\downarrow$brain volume
    - Astrocytes lose intracellular K$^+$ and osmolytes (mainly organic solutes) → allow cells to lose water and have the same osmolality as plasma, without a large $\uparrow$ in cell volume
  - Once the brain is adapted to chronic hyponatraemia, the rate of correction is extremely important:
    - In contrast, if hyponatraemia occurred rapidly (e.g. acute water intoxication in a marathon runner, ecstasy users), the patient is unlikely to develop ODS as cerebral adaptation is at an early stage
  - Rapid correction of hyponatraemia $\uparrow$plasma osmolality → cell shrinkage (as organic osmolytes cannot be quickly replaced) compared to rate of fluid loss from the cell
  - The mechanism for rapid $\downarrow$ in brain volume causing demyelination is not entirely understood:
    - A proposed theory is that $\uparrow$Na$^+$ and K$^+$ entering the cell → $\uparrow$intracellular [cation] prior to organic [osmolyte] → directly injure and induce astrocyte apoptosis → disrupt myelin-producing oligodendrocytes
    - Demyelination occurs primarily in areas of the brain that are slowest in reaccumulating osmolytes after rapid correction, such as the pons
- Cause: commonly iatrogenic due to overly rapid correction of chronic **hyponatraemia**. A useful rhyme to help remember goes: 'From low to high, your pons will die'
- Predisposing conditions: **alcoholism**, liver disease, malnutrition and SIADH

- Risk factors: serum Na$^+$ <120 mmol/l, $\uparrow$duration of hyponatraemia and $\uparrow$rapid rate of correction

EPIDEMIOLOGY

- Incidence is unknown
- ODS occurs in ♀ > ♂

PRESENTATION

- Typically delayed for 2–6 days after overly rapid elevation of serum Na$^+$ concentration
- Leads to features that are often irreversible or only partially reversible:
  - Prominent features: **spastic quadriparesis**, **pseudobulbar palsy** (dysarthria, dysphagia)
  - If severe enough → acute bilateral paralysis – **'locked-in syndrome'**, when the patient is awake but cannot move or verbally communicate

INVESTIGATIONS

- Bloods: Na$^+$, serum osmolality; it is important to continuously monitor these paramaeters, initially every 2–3 h
- CT head: shows low attenuation at the lower pons
- MRI brain (T2 weighted): shows intense symmetrical demyelination in the pons

MANAGEMENT

- Supportive management only, there is no cure
- Patients who survive ODS require extensive and prolonged neurorehabilitation
- Prevention is key: chronic hyponatraemia must be corrected with saline gradually over >48 h to avoid ODS:
  - The change in Na$^+$ must not exceed 8 mmol/l in the first 24 h and **18 mmol/l in the first 48 h**
- If the patient is at high risk of developing ODS (see predisposing conditions), consider desmopressin concurrently with saline:
  - By repeatedly administering desmopressin → induces state of iatrogenic SIADH → prevents water diuresis that can abruptly $\uparrow$Na$^+$ levels. Intervention should be done under senior supervision

COMPLICATIONS

Aspiration pneumonia, deep vein thrombosis

PROGNOSIS

ODS has a 50% mortality

PARKINSON'S DISEASE

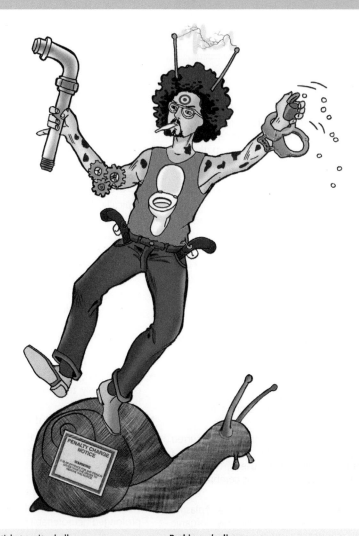

A snail has a parking ticket on its shell	**Parkinson's disease**
A man has multiple black pigmented spots on his skin	**Neuronal death in substantia nigra** Nigra (Latin) for black
He has a picture of a loo on his vest	**Lewy body** Loo-ey boy
He is smoking cannabis	**Dopamine** Smoking cannabis can be colloquially called dope
He is popping pills with his left hand, which is handcuffed	**Pill-rolling tremor, encephalitis** Handcuff sounds like 'encep'halitis
His right hand is holding a lead pipe	**Lead pipe rigidity**
His right elbow is made out of cog-wheels	**Cogwheeling**
He is falling backwards onto the snail	**Postural instability, bradykinesia** Snail = bradykinesia
He has an expressionless face	**Masked facies**
He has a target sign above his nose	**Positive glabellar reflex** 'Glabella' is the skin area above the nose
He has 2 guns inside his front trouser pockets	**'Gunslinger' pose**
There are 2 electrodes sticking out of his head	**DBS**

PARKINSON'S DISEASE

DEFINITION

An idiopathic, hypokinetic neurodegenerative disorder of dopamine-secreting neurons in the substantia nigra

AETIOLOGY

- Pathophysiology: the precise mechanisms is unknown; **loss of dopaminergic neurons in the pars compacta of the substantia nigra** → ↓dopamine in the striatum, causing disinhibition of the indirect pathway and ↓activation of the direct pathway → ↑inhibition of cortical motor areas. Surviving neurons accumulate α-synuclein (**Lewy bodies**) → neurotoxicity in the substantia nigra. Patients are symptomatic after 80% neuronal loss
- Tremor due to loss of ACh inhibition (↓**dopamine** → ↑ACh → ↑neuronal muscle activity)
- Parkinsonism: any condition that presents with cardinal movement abnormalities (**T**remor, **R**igidity, **A**kinesia and **P**ostural instability; 'TRAP'). If the cause is idiopathic it is known as PD
- Consider Parkinson's plus syndrome if TRAP + additional features are present, e.g.:
  - Cerebellar signs → multiple system atrophy
  - Impaired vertical gaze → progressive supranuclear palsy
  - Cirrhosis/liver failure → Wilson's disease
  - Other causes: **viral encephalitis**, repeated head injury, CO poisoning and MPTP ('frozen addict syndrome')

EPIDEMIOLOGY

- 1–2% of >60 y/o have PD
- Incidence is 20/100,000 per year
- It is the second most common neurodegenerative disease (after AD)

PRESENTATION

- Initial presentation may be unilateral → progresses bilaterally (over the course of ~10 years):
  - Drug-induced Parkinsonism: symptoms present bilaterally, rigidity and resting tremor are uncommon
- Positive motor:
  - Resting **'pill-rolling' tremor** (4–6 Hz); initially unilateral. Subsides with activity
  - Re-emergent tremor: re-emerges with static posture following a movement
  - Rigidity: **lead pipe** and **'cogwheeling'** (due to the combination of rigidity and tremor)
    - ↑Rigidity by asking the patient to perform an action in the opposite limb – contralateral synkinesis
- Negative motor:

- **Bradykinesia**: slowness to movement with shuffling gait (slow, small amplitude movements)
- **Masked facies**
- Reflexes:
  - **+ve glabellar reflex** (repeated glabella tapping does not diminish the blinking response)
  - **Postural instability** (loss of postural reflexes: difficulty in remaining balanced)
- Stooped posture due to generalised flexion: elbows are in flexion, known as the **'gunslinger' pose** (as the patient looks like an old western cowboy, holding onto both guns in his pockets)
- Loss of associated arm swing when walking (an early sign)
- Micrographia (handwriting becomes smaller and spidery)
- Psychiatric: depression, cognitive impairment (including psychosis)

INVESTIGATIONS

- Clinically diagnosed; using 2/4 cardinal 'TRAP' features
- L-DOPA trial: improvement of symptoms confirms the diagnosis and rules out Parkinson's plus syndromes (progressive supranuclear palsy, multiple system atrophy, etc.)
- CT/DaTSCAN: CT rules out other causes, DaTSCAN shows a reduction in dopamine transporter density in the striatum
- Definitive diagnosis → autopsy: histology shows **Lewy bodies**

MANAGEMENT

- Mainstay: L-DOPA with carbidopa (inhibits peripheral metabolism of L-DOPA by DOPA decarboxylase)
- Other adjuncts: dopamine agonists (e.g. ropinirole, pramipexole); these drugs are also effective as monotherapy in mild PD. MAO/COMT-inhibitors (↓dopamine breakdown), amantadine (↑dopamine release)
- Anticholinergics: have a modest effect in reducing tremor
- If medical therapy fails, surgical pallidotomy or **DBS**

COMPLICATIONS

- On-off motor fluctuations
- Lewy body dementia: fluctuating attention, visual hallucinations, ↑neuroleptic sensitivity

PROGNOSIS

- Gradually progressive: mean duration is 15 years
- Optimal treatment can delay disability by up to 10 years

POST-HERPETIC NEURALGIA

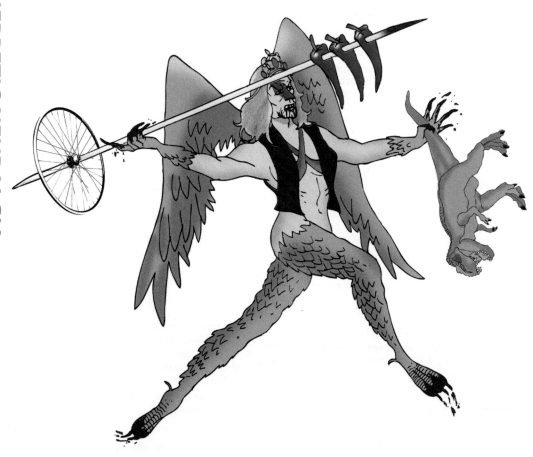

An old-aged harpy	**Post-herpetic neuralgia, old age**
She has a pink hue to her right forehead and nose, and is wearing a 3-gemmed tiara	**Dermatomal distribution (V1), trigeminal nerve**
On her left hand she is holding four fingers up; she looks in pain	**Pain persists >4 months**
She is holding a dinosaur by its tail with her gripped left thumb	**Allodynia** Allo-dynia = dino-saur
She is ready to throw a javelin	**Pregabalin**
Skewered on the tip of the javelin, there are chilli peppers	**Capsaicin**
On the javelin, there is a bicycle wheel	**Acyclovir** A cycle wheel = acyclovir

POST-HERPETIC NEURALGIA

DEFINITION

Pain confined to a dermatomal distribution after resolution of a shingles rash

AETIOLOGY

- Pathophysiology: herpes zoster presents initially with a painful vesicular eruption in a **dermatomal distribution**. The vesicular eruption resolves but in PHN the pain continues, due to destruction (via haemorrhagic inflammation) of the sensory ganglion neurons (e.g. dorsal root, **trigeminal** or geniculate ganglia)
- PHN occurs in 15% of cases after resolution of vesicular lesions
- Timeline of pain is associated with herpes zoster infection:
  - Acute herpetic neuralgia: pain preceding or accompanying the rash. It persists for up to 30 days from onset
  - Subacute herpetic neuralgia: pain persists beyond the rash healing. It resolves within 4 months of onset
  - PHN: pain persisting beyond 4 months from the initial rash onset
- Risk factors: **old age**, greater acute pain, greater rash severity

EPIDEMIOLOGY

- Incidence varies with age:
  - 60–69 y: 60%
  - >70 y: 75%

PRESENTATION

- **Pain persists >4 months** in the region of the cutaneous outbreak of herpes zoster (after resolution of the eruption)
- Distribution risk: **trigeminal (typically V$_1$)** > brachial plexus > thoracic (especially T4–T6) > cervical > lumbar > sacral
- Constant deep ache/burning, intermittently spontaneous stabbing pain, with **allodynia** (pain from non-noxious stimuli)
- Debilitating pain: impaired sleep, ↓appetite, ↓libido, depression

INVESTIGATIONS

- Clinical diagnosis
- No specific investigations are indicated

MANAGEMENT

- General advice: wear loose clothing. Use 'cling-film'/plastic wound dressings to protect sensitive areas
- Analgesia: follow the analgesic ladder; start with paracetamol or a paracetamol/codeine combination. If not sufficient consider:
  - Tricyclic antidepressants (off-licence): for moderate to severe pain:
    - Use cautiously in the elderly due to risk of anticholinergic effects
  - Gabapentin/**pregabalin** (licensed): start low and titrate up
  - **Capsaicin** (topical/patch): derived from chilli peppers; works by initially causing pain due to activation of nociceptive neurons, but over time depletes and prevents the accumulation of substance P (a nociceptive neurotransmitter) leading to pain insensitivity
  - Topical lidocaine: a Cochrane review found limited evidence for effectiveness
- Antiviral agents: early treatment with **acyclovir** → ↓herpetic neuralgia pain, duration and incidence of PHN:
  - Longer-acting famciclovir and valaciclovir are ↑effective
- VZV vaccine: shown to reduce the incidence of herpes zoster, thus reducing PHN incidence:
  - If the patient later develops PHN, the vaccine has been shown to reduce the severity and duration
- If the pain is refractory to the above measures, consider intrathecal glucocorticoid injections:
  - Note, not useful for PHN involving the trigeminal nerve
- Steroids have not been shown to reduce the incidence of PHN

COMPLICATIONS

Intractable pain

PROGNOSIS

- Most patients experience slow improvement over a long time
- A minority fail to show improvement, despite medical treatment

STROKE

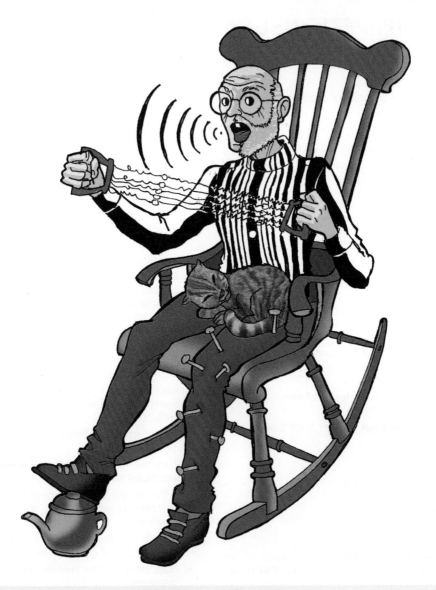

A man is wearing a striped top, representing the Doppler effect	**Stroke, Doppler** Stroke sounds like 'stripe'
He is trying hard to pull the chest expander to create tension	**Hypertension**
He is an old man	**Elderly**
He has weakness in his left arm and feels no pain from the nails in his lower limb	**Contralateral weakness/sensory loss**
His eyes show an inability to view his left visual field	**Homonymous hemianopia**
He cannot comprehend the left side of this body, indicated by him forgetting to shave the left side of his face	**Hemispatial neglect**
A cat is lying on his lap	**CT head**
He is shouting, creating sound waves	**Echo**
His foot is resting on a teapot	**tPA** tP = teapot

STROKE

DEFINITION

The sudden onset of a focal neurological deficit due to a vascular cause, lasting >24 hours

AETIOLOGY

- Pathophysiology: sudden ↓ in blood supply → severely ischaemic neurons, surrounded by an ischaemic penumbra (oedematous, viable, ischaemic neurons that are salvageable with optimal treatment). Oedematous as hypoxia → ↓ATP to manage the Na^+/K^+ -ATPase pump → vasogenic oedema
- Ischaemic (80%):
  - Atherosclerosis: thrombus formation
  - Emboli: AF, carotid stenosis, septic emboli (due to infective endocarditis)
  - Lacunar infarct: occlusion of penetrating arteries that supply deep brain structures, 2° to chronic HTN
  - Systemic hypoperfusion: global ischaemia; affects watershed areas (between major cerebral arteries)
- Haemorrhagic (20%):
  - Intracerebral: rupture of small microaneurysms (Charcot–Bouchard aneurysms); 2° to chronic HTN
  - Subarachnoid: see Subarachnoid haemorrhage
- Risk factors are the same as those for MI: **hypertension** (the single greatest risk factor), diabetes, hyperlipidaemia and smoking

EPIDEMIOLOGY

- Stroke is common in the **elderly**
- Incidence: 2/1000 per year
- The third most common cause of death in the developed world
- Most occur in the morning: the change from low to high BP on waking can dislodge an embolism

PRESENTATION

- Anterior circulation (presentation is according to which arteries are affected):
  - ACA: contralateral leg paresis and sensory loss
  - MCA: >90% of cases (as a thrombus easily passes from the carotids into the MCA):
    - **Contralateral weakness/sensory loss** of face and arm
    - **Homonymous hemianopia**/quadrantopia; eyes deviate towards the side of the lesion
    - Aphasia if the dominant hemisphere is affected; **hemispatial neglect** if the non-dominant hemisphere is affected
- Posterior circulation (presentation is according to which arteries are affected):
  - PCA: homonymous hemianopia/quandrantopia with macular sparing, prosopagnosia (only if bilateral)
  - Basilar: cranial nerve pathologies, impaired consciousness, locked-in syndrome

- AICA: vertigo, ataxia, ipsilateral deafness and ipsilateral facial weakness
- PICA: see Wallenberg syndrome
- Lacunar: pure contralateral sensory loss (if the thalamus is affected) or pure motor loss (if the posterior limb of the internal capsule is affected)
- Intracerebral haemorrhage (due to ↑ICP): headache, meningism, N&V, seizures, altered level of consciousness

INVESTIGATIONS

- Best initial test: **CT head**, no contrast (differentiates ischaemic from haemorrhagic stroke)
- Most accurate test: MRI; identifies early ischaemic changes. 95% sensitive for ischaemic stroke in 24 h
- ECG/**echo**: used if embolic stroke is suspected (AF: start anticoagulation; mitral stenosis: valvuloplasty):
  - If 2° to AF, haemorrhage must be ruled out and 14 d elapsed before starting anticoagulation. LMWH cover is given in the interim
- USS carotid **Doppler** (>70% occlusion → carotid endarterectomy)
- If young (<50 y/o): thrombophilia screen (for hypercoagulable states), ESR/autoantibodies (for vasculitis)

MANAGEMENT

- Admit to stroke unit. Maintain hydration, blood glucose, O_2 saturation within normal limits:
  - If ischaemic, do not ↓BP in the acute phase; it is necessary to maintain perfusion to ischaemic penumbra
- Ischaemic stroke + <4.5 h from presentation → **tPA** (e.g. alteplase)
- Ischaemic stroke + >4.5 h from presentation or thrombolysis C/I → 300 mg aspirin. If intolerant → clopidogrel 75 mg
- Haemorrhagic stroke → aim therapy to manage ↑ICP (mannitol, antihypertensives) and control seizures
- MDT involvement; calculate the NIHSS score (assesses the severity of acute stroke; this informs treatment)
- Manage risk factors; if cholesterol >3.5 mmol commence a statin (wait 48 h due to risk of haemorrhagic transformation)
- If a single instance of stroke → the patient cannot drive for 1 month

COMPLICATIONS

- Cerebral oedema (↑ICP), aspiration pneumonia, malnutrition
- Death (↑ with haemorrhagic stroke)

PROGNOSIS

- Mortality: 20% in 1st 2 months, then roughly 10% per year thereafter
- <40% of patients make a full recovery

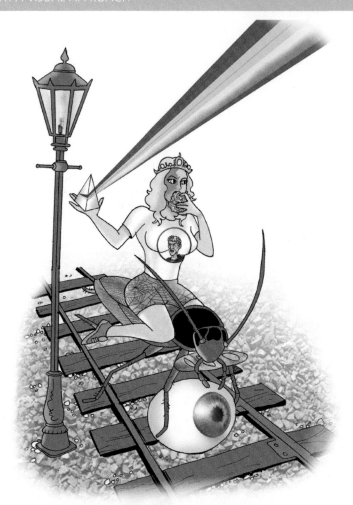

A woman is wearing a blue skirt with web patterning	**Sturge–Weber syndrome** Sturge loosely sounds like 'skirt'
She is gnawing on snack mix	***GNAQ* gene** 'GNAQ' loosely rhymes with 'snack'
The woman is riding a large cockroach	**Roach classification**
Nearly half of the woman's face has a red stain	**Port-wine stain**
She is wearing 3-gemmed tiara	**Trigeminal nerve** 3-gem = 'trigem'inal nucleus
The cockroach is squashing an eyeball	**Glaucoma** Raised intraocular pressure
The woman is wearing a T-shirt depicting Julius Caesar	**Epilepsy** Caesar = seizure
The woman's eyes can only view half of her visual field	**Homonymous hemianopia**
The cockroach is on top of train-tracks	**Tram-track calcifications**
The cockroach is eating a baguette	**Carbamazepine** Baguette = carbs = carbamazepine
Next to the woman there is a lantern post	**Latanoprost**
In her right hand she is holding a prism that is splitting light	**Pulsed dye laser** Prism forming a stream of light like a laser of different colours (dye)

STURGE–WEBER SYNDROME

DEFINITION

A neurocutaneous disorder classically affecting the cranial nerve V_1 distribution, with associated angiomatous brain malformations

AETIOLOGY

- Pathophysiology: activating a mutation of the **GNAQ gene** → abnormal growth of neural crest derivatives (mesoderm/ectoderm) and inhibition of apoptosis. Normally, during embryology a vascular plexus develops around the neural tube, then regresses. Inhibition of apoptosis causes persistence of these vascular tissues → angiomas (benign blood vessel tumours) of the leptomeninges, face and ipsilateral eye
- Involvement of one or all three; classified by '**Roach classification**':
  - Type 1: both facial and leptomeningeal angiomas: may have glaucoma
  - Type 2: facial angioma alone: many have glaucoma
  - Type 3: isolated leptomeningeal angioma: usually no glaucoma
- Cause: congenital; non-inherited (somatic)

EPIDEMIOLOGY

- Incidence: 1/50,000 live births
- ♂ and ♀ are equally affected

PRESENTATION

- **Port-wine stain** (*aka* cutaneous angioma):
  - Seen at birth; typically present on the forehead and upper eyelid. They are usually light pink in colour
  - Development follows the embryological pattern of facial development rather than the neuro-developmental pattern (it just so happens to be in the **distribution of the ophthalmic/maxillary branch of the trigeminal nerve**)
  - If it affects the entire V_1 distribution: strong predictor of underlying neurological and/or ocular disorders
  - Darkens with age to a deep red, 'port-wine' appearance
- **Glaucoma**: commonly on the side ipsilateral to the port-wine stain
- **Epilepsy**: focal tonic–clonic seizures occur typically in the first year. Due to leptomeningeal involvement:

- Seen in up to 90% of patients
- Occur on the opposite side to the port-wine stain
- Can become generalised and evolve into drop attacks, myoclonic or infantile spasms
- Can be accompanied by hemiparesis
- Visual field defects: typically **homonymous hemianopia**; due to leptomeningeal involvement affecting the optic tracts
- Neuropsychological development: intellectual disability and behavioural problems

INVESTIGATIONS

- Diagnosis is suspected when a newborn has a facial port-wine birthmark
- Best initial and most accurate test: MRI + gadolinium; checks for involvement of leptomeninges and brain structures:
  - −ve brain MRI at 1 y/o can reliably exclude the presence of leptomeningeal lesions
- CT head: shows characteristic '**tram-track calcifications' sign**, i.e. cortical calcifications between the pia and arachnoid mater of the opposing gyri

MANAGEMENT

- Symptomatic only
- Medical: **carbamazepine** for seizure control; **latanoprost** (a prostaglandin analogue) for ↓IOP in glaucoma
- Surgical: **pulsed dye laser** for the port-wine stain. Effective in infants <6 m/o:
  - If there is refractory epilepsy → hemispherectomy
- Ocular monitoring: for glaucoma
- Cosmetic camouflage cream: conceals the port-wine stain

COMPLICATIONS

Status epilepticus, developmental delay

PROGNOSIS

- Prognosis is dependent on the extent of leptomeningeal malformation
- It is also affected by age of onset of seizures and whether seizure control can be achieved

SUBACUTE COMBINED DEGENERATION

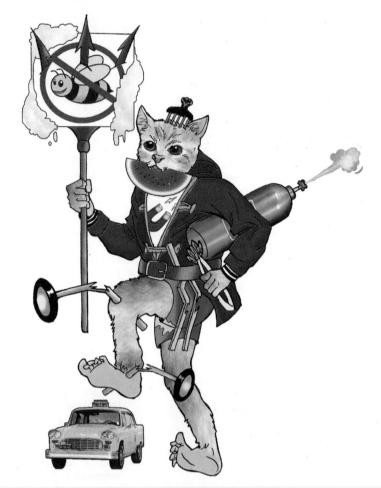

A cute cat with a comb lodged in its hair	**Subacute combined degeneration** Suba'cute' = cat; combined = comb
It is holding a 'no-bees' poster	**Posterior columns, vitamin B$_{12}$ deficiency** Poster = posterior; B$_{12}$ deficiency = bees not allowed
It is wearing a red coat and holding celery in its left hand	**Lateral corticospinal tracts, dorsal spinocerebellar tracts** Cortico = coat; spino'cere' = celery spine (stalk)
It is eating a watermelon slice	**Methylmalonic acid** 'Malon'ic = melon
Underneath its left armpit is an N$_2$O canister leaking gas	**N$_2$O exposure**
There is a broken tuning fork underneath its belt at the waist	**Loss of vibration sense**
It is adopting a stomping position, about to crush a toy taxi	**Stomping gait, ataxia**
The cat's feet are fanning upwards	**Babinski sign +ve (UMN lesion)**
Through the cat's left knee and left ankle, there are broken tendon hammers	**Absent knee jerks and ankle jerks (LMN lesion)**
It is holding a demon trident	**Dementia**
A wet patch can be seen near the groin region	**Urinary incontinence**
There are foam bubbles hanging from the poster board	**Folic acid** Fo-am = Fo-lic
The cat has a picture of a magnet on its T-shirt	**MRI**

SUBACUTE COMBINED DEGENERATION

DEFINITION

A degeneration of the **posterior columns, lateral corticospinal tracts** and **dorsal spinocerebellar tracts**, commonly as a result of vitamin B_{12} deficiency

AETIOLOGY

- Pathophysiology: vitamin B_{12} is a co-factor for methylmalonyl-CoA mutase to convert **methylmalonic acid** to succinyl CoA (which is incorporated into the myelin sheath). B_{12} deficiency results in ↑levels of methylmalonic acid, which impairs spinal cord myelination. The dorsal columns and lateral corticospinal tracts are heavily myelinated, hence they are greatly affected
- Gradual causes: **vitamin B_{12} deficiency** (most common), vitamin E deficiency or Friedreich's ataxia
- Acutely: **N_2O exposure** causing B_{12} deficiency iatrogenically (e.g. anaesthesia) or recreationally ('whippets'):
  - N_2O oxidises the cobalt atom of B_{12} → inactivates B_{12}'s co-factor function

EPIDEMIOLOGY

- Peak age: 60 y/o
- Incidence (of pernicious anaemia): 1/10,000

PRESENTATION

- Early features: loss of fine touch and **vibration sense** (paraesthesia) and conscious proprioception (**ataxia**):
  - Many present with falls at night due to a combination of ataxia and reduced vision in the dark:
    - May adopt a **stomping gait**; forceful walking ↓sensory information from the legs
- Classical triad: **extensor plantars** (UMN), **absent knee jerks** (LMN) and **absent ankle jerks** (LMN)
- Peripheral neuropathy (variable reversibility): usually symmetrical, affecting lower limbs > upper limbs
- Cerebral (common, reversible with B_{12} therapy) – confusion, delirium, **dementia**
- Cranial nerves: rare – optic atrophy
- Late features: severe weakness, clonus, paraplegia, and even faecal and **urinary incontinence**:
  - Prolonged B_{12} deficiency (>3 months) leads to irreversible nervous system damage
- Pain and temperature may remain intact even in severe cases, as the spinothalamic tracts are preserved

INVESTIGATIONS

- Best initial test: B_{12} levels:
  - Transcobalamin; acts to bind B_{12} and is also an acute-phase reactant. In the presence of stress/infection → ↑transcobalamin → ↑B_{12} levels even though total B_{12} is low
- Most accurate test: ↑**methylmalonic acid** levels
- Other bloods:
  - FBC (↓Hb, ↑MCV):
    - It is possible to have neurological disease without anaemia (seen in 28%)
  - **Folic acid** (if deficient, must be managed after the B_{12} deficiency has been corrected; see below)
  - Blood film: hypersegmented neutrophils
- Antibodies: intrinsic factor antibody (100% specific for pernicious anaemia)
- **MRI brain**: symmetrical bilateral high signal within the dorsal columns

MANAGEMENT

- Best initial treatment: IM vitamin B_{12} injection (initially 1 mg repeated 5 times at intervals of 2–3 days; maintenance dose 1 mg every 3 months):
  - B_{12} therapy improves peripheral nerve damage but the improvement in spinal cord function is not always significant
  - Monitor K^+ levels: starting B_{12} replacement → ↑haematopoiesis → K^+ internalisation → can ↓K^+ in the blood
- If folic acid and vitamin B_{12} deficient, the vitamin B_{12} deficiency must be treated first to avoid precipitating subacute combined degeneration:
  - Giving folic acid first will turn the remaining B_{12} into methylcobalamin. This means B_{12} cannot act as a co-factor for methylmalonyl-CoA mutase to convert methylmalonic acid → succinyl CoA = poor myelination

COMPLICATIONS

Irreversible ataxia, dementia, spastic paralysis and urinary incontinence

PROGNOSIS

Vitamin B_{12} therapy results in partial to full recovery, depending on the duration and extent of any neurodegeneration

SUBARACHNOID HAEMORRHAGE

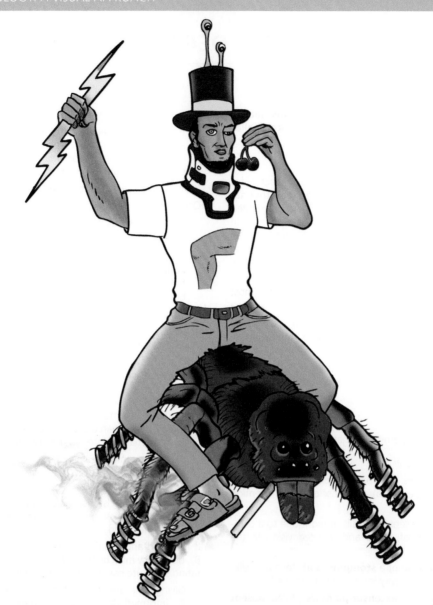

A man is riding a tarantula that is smoking a cigarette	**Subarachnoid haemorrhage, smoking** Tarantula = Arachnoid
The man is about to eat some berries	**Berry aneurysms**
He has 'martian' antennae sticking out of his hat	**Marfan's syndrome** Marfan sounds similar to Martian
He is holding a thunderbolt	**Thunderclap headache**
He is wearing a neck brace	**Neck stiffness**
His left eye is in the 'down and out' position with ptosis	**CN III palsy**
He is wearing a sandal on his right foot	**Sentinel bleed** Sandal loosely sounds like sentinel
His hat has a yellow ribbon	**Xanthochromia**
The tarantula's legs are covered with coils	**Endovascular coiling**
His T-Shirt has a picture of a bent knee	**Nimodipine** Knee-modipine

SUBARACHNOID HAEMORRHAGE

DEFINITION
An arterial bleed into the subarachnoid space. It may be spontaneous or 2° to trauma (the commonest cause)

AETIOLOGY
- Pathophysiology: aneurysmal **SAH** occur due to rupture of **saccular 'berry' aneurysms**:
  - Commonly occur at branching points of the circle of Willis vessels, as there is lack of tunica media here. Ischaemia results 2° to vasospasm → brain damage
- Spontaneous SAH is a type of stroke; the commonest cause is a ruptured aneurysm (85%)
- Associations: trauma, genetic conditions (**Marfan's syndrome**, ADPKD)
- 'Mycotic' aneurysms: seen in infective endocarditis; infective emboli lodge commonly in the MCA and damage the arterial wall
- Risk factors: hypertension, **smoking**, drug abuse (cocaine and amphetamines), COCP, pregnancy

EPIDEMIOLOGY
- Annual incidence: 1/10,000
- Peak onset: 55–60 y/o

PRESENTATION
- Abrupt-onset, intensely painful **'thunderclap'** **headache** (the worst headache of their life; up to 97% sensitive, 25% specific):
  - Classically described as 'blow to the head with a bat'; mainly occipital
- Altered level of consciousness; graded using the WFNS grading system
- Meningism: **neck stiffness**, photophobia, N&V, +ve Kernig's/Brudzinski's sign
- ↑ICP signs: papilloedema, cranial nerve VI palsy
- Focal neurological signs (due to expanding aneurysm/intracerebral haematoma compressing on adjacent structures):
  - Basilar/posterior communicating artery aneurysm → **CN III palsy**
  - Intracavernous sinus carotid aneurysms → ophthalmoplegia (III, IV and VI) and/or facial pain (V_1 nerve)
  - ICA/anterior communicating artery aneurysm → visual field defects (optic chiasm), hypopituitarism (pituitary stalk)
  - MCA aneurysm → hemiparesis (motor cortex/internal capsule)
- Warning headache, aka **'sentinel bleed'**: precedes SAH in >50% of patients:
  - 30–60% of patients with SAH give a history suggestive of sentinel bleed within the past 3 weeks

- Thought to be the result of small leaks prior to rupture. Resolve rapidly with no other symptoms
- Cardiovascular: due to ↑ICP → Cushing's response (HTN, ↓HR, irregular respirations):
  - If a murmur is auscultated, consider infective endocarditis as a possible SAH cause (mycotic aneurysm)

INVESTIGATIONS
- Blood: FBC, U&E, clotting screen
- Best initial test: CT head with no contrast; hyperdensity is seen in the subarachnoid space. >95% sensitivity in severe SAH. If CT is not diagnostic (seen in 2%), an LP should be performed
- Most accurate test: LP; it is bloody or **xanthochromic** (yellow; due to Hb breakdown):
  - LP may be falsely −ve in the first 6–12 hours (xanthochromia has not yet developed)
  - If alert + no focal signs → LP. If unconscious or with focal signs → no LP; refer as soon as possible
- If normal WBC:RBC in CSF ratio = SAH, if ↑↑WBC:RBC, suspect meningitis
- CT head angiography: locates the source of bleeding; it is performed if the patient is a candidate for surgery
- Gold standard test: digital subtraction 4-vessel angiography, a fluoroscopic technique

MANAGEMENT
- Acute: admit to ITU, obtain a neurosurgical review
- Definitive treatment: **endovascular coiling**; this blocks blood flow into the aneurysm. It is superior to surgical clipping
- Prevent vasospasm: **nimodipine** (a CCB) → improves neurological outcome
- Treat hydrocephalus: use a lumbar drain or serial LPs

COMPLICATIONS
- Hydrocephalus; either non-communicating (CSF blockage due to a blood clot) or communicating (arachnoid villi/meninges damage, due to haemorrhage)
- Re-bleeding, stroke (2° to vasospasm)

PROGNOSIS
- 15% mortality before reaching hospital; overall, 50% mortality
- 30% of survivors have moderate to severe disability

SUBDURAL HAEMATOMA

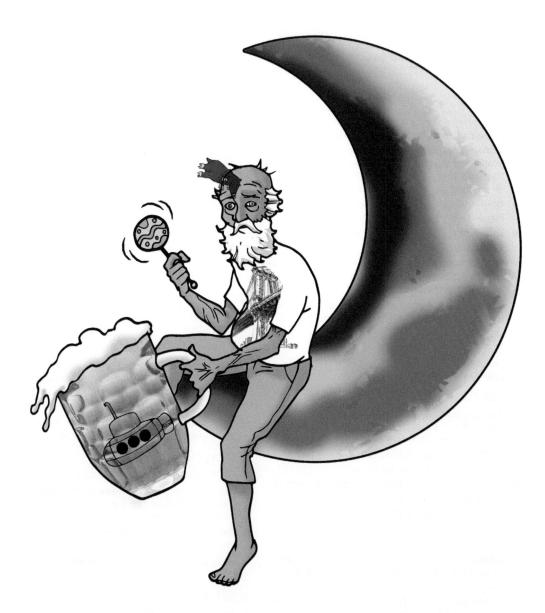

A submarine is submerged in a beer glass	Subdural haematoma
His is wearing a T-shirt of a bridge	Bridging veins
He is an old man with a beer belly and is holding a large beer	Elderly, alcoholic
He is shaking a baby rattler	Shaken baby syndrome
His left arm is weak (he cannot hold the beer up), and his left leg is dangling	Contralateral hemiparesis
His right pupil is very dilated	Ipsilateral dilated pupil
He is sitting on a waxing crescent moon	Crescent-shaped concave hyperdensity
A mole is burrowing into his skull	Burr hole

SUBDURAL HAEMATOMA

DEFINITION
Occurs typically following head trauma; SDH leads to rupture of bridging veins and slow accumulation of blood between the dura and arachnoid membranes

AETIOLOGY
- Pathophysiology: cerebral veins (*aka* **bridging veins**) drain into dural venous sinuses. If the position of the dura and brain suddenly shift (e.g. trauma causing sudden acceleration/deceleration) → shearing forces rupture the bridging veins. Slow venous bleeding (↓pressure → haematoma develops gradually compared to extradural haematoma)
- Usually occurs following trauma leading to head injury:
  - Can occur spontaneously (unrelated to trauma): e.g. due to hypertension, arteriovenous malformations or dural metastases
- Risk factors: cerebral atrophy → ↑subdural space (**elderly and alcoholics**), blunt trauma, anticoagulant therapy
- In a paediatric patient if coupled with retinal haemorrhages → consider as **shaken baby syndrome** until proven otherwise

EPIDEMIOLOGY
- Acute: ↑young patients/major trauma. ↑common than extradural haemorrhage
- Chronic: ↑in elderly; 1–5/100,000. Peak incidence: >80 y/o

PRESENTATION
- Timeframe: acutely: <72 h; subacutely: 3–20 days; chronic: >3 weeks
- Acute: headaches, altered mental status, focal neurological signs (**contralateral hemiparesis, ipsilateral dilated pupil**):
  - Posterior fossa SDH presents with symptoms of ↑ICP (headache, vomiting, anisocoria, dysphagia, cranial nerve palsies and meningism); presentation is similar to most space-occupying lesions in this location
  - Can present with a lucid interval and progressive neurological decline to coma
- Chronic: gait disturbances, psychiatric symptoms; may present as pseudodementia in the elderly:
  - Global deficits (i.e. disturbances of consciousness) are more common than focal deficits (i.e. after acute SDH)

- Symptoms may not become evident until weeks after the initial injury
- Seizures may be occasionally seen
- Bitemporal chronic SDH: may present with proximal, painless intermittent paraparesis
- Especially if the patient is elderly/alcoholic, SDH should be considered, even if there is no history of trauma

INVESTIGATIONS
- Bloods: FBC, U&E (particularly Na⁺; due to cerebral salt wasting), clotting screen (to correct any coagulopathy)
- Best initial test: CT head; shows a **crescent-shaped concave hyperdensity** acutely (isodense subacutely, hypodense chronically). It is possible to have mixed density (a new haemorrhage into an old collection; 'acute on chronic' SDH):
  - Crosses suture lines (as the subdural space is not bound by sutural ligaments)
  - Cannot cross the midline due to the cerebral falx/cerebellar tentorium (whereas structures can be crossed in an extradural haematoma)
- Most accurate test: MRI brain; sensitivity for isodense/small SDHs (easily missed)

MANAGEMENT
- Severe trauma: immobilisation of the cervical spine, trauma team alerted
- Surgical evacuation (**burr hole** or craniotomy) if symptomatic or ↑in size. ICP monitoring devices may be placed *in situ*
- If chronic, conservative management with serial imaging → subdural blood may regress spontaneously

COMPLICATIONS
- ↑ICP, cerebral oedema
- Mass effect (transtentorial, uncal), seizures

PROGNOSIS
- Acute: mortality rates are 50–90%, largely due to underlying brain injury
- Chronic: better outcomes than acute SDHs

SYRINGOMYELIA

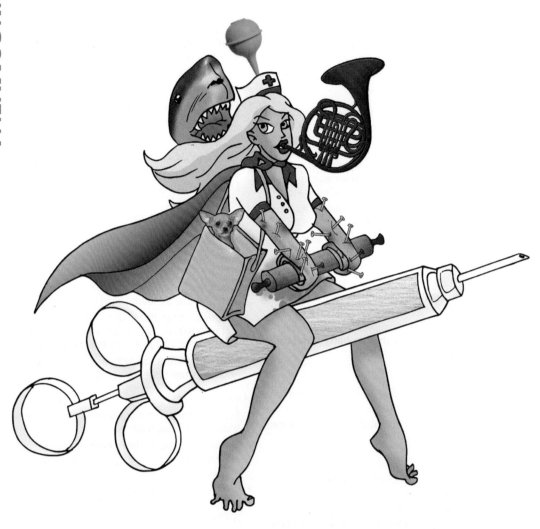

A nurse is riding a large syringe	**Syringomyelia**
She has nails, cuts and bruises on her arms but feels no pain	**Bilateral loss of pain and temperature sensation, scars, bruises and ulcers**
She is playing a blue French horn	**Horner's syndrome**
She has a handbag with a chihuahua inside	**Arnold–Chiari malformation**
She is wearing an old style nurse's cape	**Cape-like distribution**
She has a shark head coming out of her hair	**Charcot joint**
Her feet are fanning upwards	**Babinski +ve (UMN sign)**
Her hands and forearm are wound around a rolling pin and very weak	**Muscle atrophy (distal → proximal)**
She has wet herself	**Bladder dysfunction**
She has a bulb syringe sticking out of her hat	**Syringobulbia**

SYRINGOMYELIA

DEFINITION
A cystic enlargement of the central canal of the spinal cord causing progressive myelopathy, initially affecting the crossed lateral spinothalamic tracts in the central part of the spinal cord

AETIOLOGY
- Pathophysiology: the syrinx (a CSF-filled cavity within the spinal cord) expands and damages the anterior white commissure of the spinothalamic tract (2nd order neurons) → **bilateral loss of pain and temperature sensation** (usually C8–T1 initially). Further expansion can compress the anterior horns causing LMN signs in the upper limb, and lateral horns, preventing sympathetic outflow (if this occurs at T1, it can cause **Horner's syndrome**):
  - Primary syringomyelia: aetiology is unknown
  - Secondary syringomyelia: intramedullary tumour, trauma (scars in the arachnoid membrane preventing CSF outflow), **Arnold–Chiari I malformation** (>70% of cases)

EPIDEMIOLOGY
- Mean age of onset: 30 y/o
- Incidence: ~8/100,000

PRESENTATION
- A slowly progressive condition as the syrinx takes time to enlarge before symptoms occur
- Localisation of the lesion: the presentation reflects the extent of the syrinx enlargement:
  - Anterior white commissure extension:
    - Dissociated sensory loss: **'cape-like' bilateral loss of pain and temperature** (arms, back and upper chest). Fine touch, vibration and proprioception are preserved (dorsal columns are intact)
    - May present with **scars, bruises** and **ulcers** on the arms and hands as no sensory arc of withdrawal reflex is present
    - **Charcot joints**: painless neuropathic arthropathies in the shoulder and neck due to **loss of pain and temperature sensation** (occur in <5%)
  - Descending corticospinal tract extension:
    - Lower limb UMN signs: spasticity, weakness, hyper-reflexia, **Babinski +ve**; due to the involvement of the descending corticospinal tracts

- Anterior horn cell extension:
  - **Muscle atrophy**: due to extension into the anterior horns of the spinal cord; begins in the hands and **progresses proximally**
- Lateral horn cells extension:
  - **Horner's syndrome**: if occurs at T1
  - Autonomic symptoms: **bladder, bowel and sexual dysfunction** can occur
- Brainstem extension (rare):
  - **Syringobulbia**; if the syrinx extends into the brainstem → nystagmus, dysphagia, trigeminal nerve sensory loss. Respiratory failure can occur (due to damage to respiratory centres in the medulla)
- Lumbar region extension:
  - Lumbar syringomyelia: leg muscle atrophy with dissociated sensory loss in the lumbar + sacral region
- Scoliosis: prior to undergoing surgery for scoliosis correction, the patient should have an MRI to exclude syringomyelia

INVESTIGATIONS
- Best initial and most accurate test: MRI spine; shows CSF accumulation within the cord (myelography is rarely used)
- CT head: rules out 2° causes of syringomyelia

MANAGEMENT
- MDT approach: PT and rehabilitation to preserve neurological function
- Teach patients to avoid damage due to absence of pain
- Definitive: syringostomy (drainage of the syrinx). A syringo-peritoneal shunt can also be used
- Decompress the Arnold–Chiari malformation

COMPLICATIONS
Pneumonia: the most common single cause of death

PROGNOSIS
- Very rarely, a syrinx may spontaneously regress
- Mortality is highest in the first 2 years after injury

TRIGEMINAL NEURALGIA

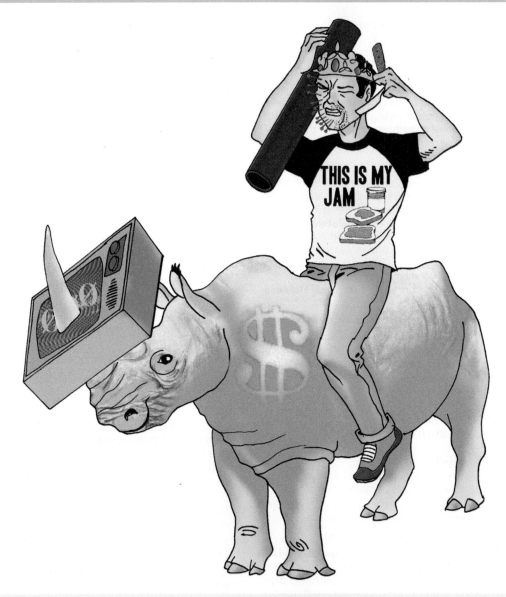

A man is riding a rhino with a large dollar symbol imprint on it	**Tic douloureux, rhizotomy** Dollar = doulour-eux
The man is in agony	**One of the most painful conditions**
He is lifting a large heavy red tube that is compressing his tiara	**Compression of trigeminal nerve by blood vessel** Tube = blood vessel, compressing on tiara (trigeminal nerve)
The rhino's horn has pierced an old-style TV	**Multiple sclerosis** A TV with 'multiple zeroes'
The man is wearing a 3-gemmed tiara, with multiple nails found distributed on the right side of his face; there are more around the jaw and fewer around the forehead	**Trigeminal nerve, $V_3 > V_2 > V_1$, stabbing pain** More nails are found in the V_3 distribution (lower jaw), than V_1 (forehead) – to depict frequently affected CN V divisions
The man is trying to shave with his left hand	**Shaving (trigger)**
Around his nose and lips, there are areas of unshaven hair	**Unshaven area on the face (trigger zone)**
He is wearing a T-shirt about bread	**Carbamazepine** Bread = 'carbs' = 'carb'amazepine

TRIGEMINAL NEURALGIA

DEFINITION

An abrupt, severe repeated electric-shock like pain in the distribution of one of the CN V divisions. Each episode typically lasts a few seconds. There may be a continuous aching pain in the background

AETIOLOGY

- Also known as **tic douloureux** ('painful tic' – as the face characteristically screws up with pain); it is considered to be **one of the most painful conditions** known to mankind
- Pathophysiology:
  - Classical TN: **compression of the trigeminal nerve at its REZ by a tortuous blood vessel** (i.e. superior cerebellar artery). Over time this wears away at the myelin sheath, increasing the likelihood of nerve excitation
  - Secondary TN: cerebellopontine angle tumour (5%), **MS** (5%):
    - MS causes demyelination plaque at the REZ, causing nerve fibre exposure and irritation
- **Divisions of trigeminal nerve** frequently affected are: $V_3 > V_2 > V_1$
- Triggers: touching the face, eating, talking, cold wind, **shaving** or applying make-up:
  - Small areas in the nasolabial fold or chin are particularly susceptible to triggering pain:
    - Ephaptic cross-talk between nerves mediating light touch and nociception may account for this

EPIDEMIOLOGY

- Annual incidence: 27/100,000
- Age: usually >50 y/o; in MS younger patients may be affected
- ♀ > ♂

PRESENTATION

- Short **stabbing pains**; extremely painful in the distribution of the affected division of CN V:

- Pain lasts seconds/minutes over days/weeks; remits for weeks/months
- Some patients with longstanding TN may have continuous dull pain present between episodes
- Almost always unilateral. If bilateral, MS should be considered as a cause
- If ♂; may have an **unshaven area on the face** (a trigger zone, which the patient avoids touching)
- A normal neurological examination is found
- Some patients may have 'pre-TN: a milder, dull, continuous pain in the jaw that can evolve into TN

INVESTIGATIONS

- A clinical diagnosis
- MRI head (with neurovascular protocol): examine REZ for compression/demyelination

MANAGEMENT

- 1st line: **carbamazepine**. Opioid analgesics are not effective
- 2nd line: baclofen, lamotrigine, amitriptyline
- Surgery (for medically resistant cases):
  - To relieve pressure on the trigeminal nerve or, conversely, to damage the nerve completely to prevent further pain
    - Microvascular decompression (of CN V) – best for classical TN
    - Rhizotomy (literally: cut nerve): gamma knife radiosurgery (produces lesions with focused gamma radiation), percutaneous balloon compression **rhizotomy**

COMPLICATIONS

Weight loss, depression – due to excruciating pain the patient has mental and physical incapacity

PROGNOSIS

Over time, pain may become ↑refractory to treatment

TUBEROUS SCLEROSIS

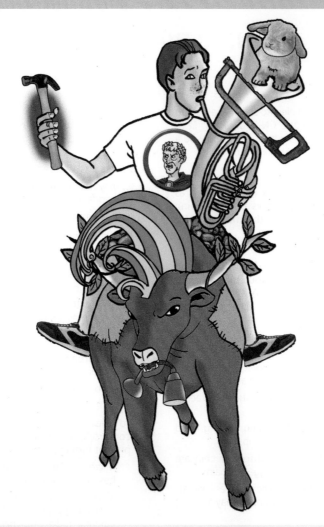

A boy is playing a large tuba	**Tuberous sclerosis, tuberin**
In his right hand, he is wielding a hammer	**Hamartoma, hamartin**
Around the horns of a bull there are ash leaves	**Ash-leaf lesions**
The boy has small red nodules around his nose	**Adenoma sebaceum**
The bull has green patch-work on its body	**Shagreen patches**
Underneath the boy's nails, there are skin lesions (best seen on his right hand)	**Subungual/periungual fibromas**
He is wearing shorts that have a coffee bean design	**Café-au-lait spots**
Cutting into the side of the tuba there is a hacksaw	**Phakomas** 'Phak' sounds like 'hack'saw
There is a rabbit sitting inside the tuba	**Rhabdomyomas** 'Rhab-bit'
The bull is holding a lamp in its mouth	**LAM (pulmonary lymphangioliomyomatosis)** LAM = Lamp
The boy is wearing a T-shirt depicting Julius Caesar	**Epilepsy** Caesar = seizure
The bull's mohawk hair resembles sea waves	**SEGA (Subependymal giant cell astrocytoma)** Sea = Sega
The handle of the hammer has a UV glow	**Wood's UV lamp**

TUBEROUS SCLEROSIS

DEFINITION
A neurocutaneous disorder with multi-system organ involvement, characterised by numerous hamartomas

AETIOLOGY
- Pathophysiology: autosomal dominant; defect in *TSC1* (on chr. 9 coding for **hamartin**) and *TSC2* (on chr. 16 coding for **tuberin**) genes. These proteins normally act synergistically to regulate cell proliferation and differentiation. Mutation leads to cell dysregulation → **hamartoma** formation (non-malignant). These can affect many organ systems:
  - Glioneuronal hamartomas are known as tubers (hence the namesake), referring to the pathological finding of thick, hardened and pale gyri in the brains of patients post mortem
- The frequency of cases due to mutations in the *TSC2* gene is higher, and is associated with a ↑severe disease progression
- Previously known as EPILOIA (epilepsy, low intelligence, adenoma sebaceum) 80–90% occur as *de novo* mutations

EPIDEMIOLOGY
- Incidence at birth: 1/5800

PRESENTATION
- Manifests with multiple hamartomas (benign, focal malformation that resemble a neoplasm in the tissue of origin):
  - Symptoms 2° to hamartomas that grow in the areas shown below
- Skin/nail manifestations:
  - **Ash-leaf** hypopigmented lesions on the trunk and extremities
  - **Adenoma sebaceum**: small red nodules; often in a malar distribution
  - **Shagreen patches** (rough papules in the lumbosacral region with orange-peel consistency)
  - **Subungual/periungual fibromas** (fibromas beneath/surrounding the nails)
  - **Café-au-lait spots** may be seen (not diagnostic)
- Retinal hamartomas; *aka* astrocytic hamartomas (or '**phakomas**')
- Heart **rhabdomyomas**:
  - Usually the first sign detected in young children. Can be picked up antenatally
  - Can regress completely or remain consistent in size
- Pulmonary involvement:

- **LAM**; commonly affects ♀. Patients present with SOB
- Neurological features:
  - Developmental delay and Intellectual disability
  - **Epilepsy** (infantile spasms or partial); due to cortical tuber formation:
    - Seen in 80%; mostly in childhood
  - **SEGA**: rare; can lead to hydrocephalus
- Renal involvement: angiomyolipomas (benign kidney hamartomas), renal cysts and renal cell carcinoma:
  - Hamartomas: usually asymptomatic in childhood. In adults they can rupture → intrarenal haemorrhage
  - Genes *TSC2* and ADPKD *PKD1* gene are contiguous on chr. 16 → mutation can cause both conditions

INVESTIGATIONS
- Diagnosis is usually clinical
- Skin lesions are enhanced under examination by **Wood's UV lamp**
- MRI: head → shows calcified tubers (glioneuronal hamartomas) within the cerebrum. Renal: best modality for renal lesions
- Fundoscopy: for retinal lesions
- Cardiac echo: for rhabdomyoma of the heart, especially in the left ventricle apex (affects >50% of patients)

MANAGEMENT
- MDT approach; symptomatic treatment only. Annual follow-up
- Conservative: developmental, psychological and behavioural assessment. Social support
- Medical: antiepileptics, such as carbamazepine; antihypertensives (in renal disease)
- Surgical: early intervention for disfiguring skin lesions and symptomatic hamartomas. Consider if refractory epilepsy
- Genetic counselling and screening of family members

COMPLICATIONS
Common causes of death are status epilepticus or bronchopneumonia

PROGNOSIS
- 30% die before 10 y/o
- 75% die before 25 y/o

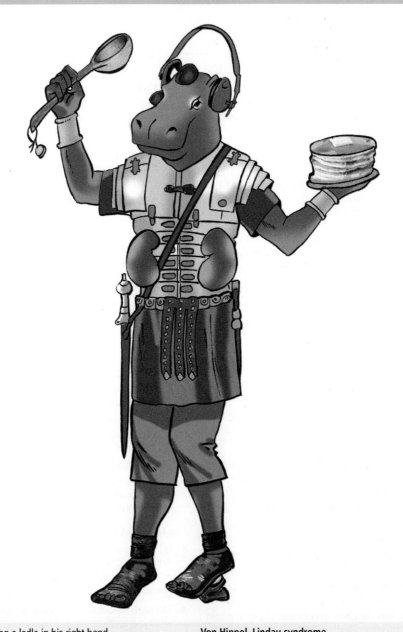

A hippo holding a ladle in his right hand	**Von Hippel–Lindau syndrome** Hippo = Hippel; ladle = Lindau
The hippo is crushing a cola can under its left foot	**Tumour suppressor gene** Can (cancer) is compressed (suppressed) under foot
It has 3 tassels hanging from around a belt	**Chromosome 3**
There are red, vascular swellings on its eye and head	**CNS and retinal haemangioblastomas**
It is wearing Roman soldier armour	**Phaeochromocytoma** Phaeo-chromo (Rome)
It has 2 large kidney-shaped impressions around his armour bilaterally	**Renal involvement: RCC and cysts**
It is holding pancakes up in its left hand	**Pancreatic tumours** Pancake = pancreatic
It is wearing earmuffs	**Hearing loss**

VON HIPPEL–LINDAU SYNDROME

DEFINITION

An heritable or acquired multi-system cancer syndrome due to a *VHL* tumour suppressor gene mutation

AETIOLOGY

- Pathophysiology: normal **VHL tumour suppressor gene** function → degrade HIF1a – a transcription factor that promotes angiogenesis. *VHL* gene mutation → ↑HIF1a activity → unregulated blood vessel growth → resulting tumours are highly vascular. 20% of cases are new mutations
- Autosomal dominant mutations of the *VHL* tumour suppressor gene (located on short arm of **chr. 3**)
- Highly penetrant: i.e. a person with the mutation is likely to develop at least one feature of VHL (*see Presentation*)
- Classification (families are classified according to the likelihood of developing phaeochromocytoma):
  - Type 1 families: low risk of phaeochromocytoma, however high risk of developing other VHL tumour types
  - Type 2 families: high risk of phaeochromocytoma with:
    - Type 2A: low risk of RCC
    - Type 2B: high risk of RCC
    - Type 2C: phaeochromocytoma with no other VHL–associated tumour

EPIDEMIOLOGY

- Age: early childhood to seventh decade
- Mean age is 27 y/o
- Incidence: 1/36,000 live births

PRESENTATION

- **CNS haemangioblastomas** (usually in the cerebellum, spinal cord or brainstem):
  - Presentation varies depending on the location: headache, ataxia, sensory loss
- **Retinal haemangioblastomas** (found in 60% of patients):
  - Commonly the first presentation
  - Usually asymptomatic. If complicated → retinal detachment, vitreous haemorrhage and vision loss
- **Phaeochromocytomas**:
  - Mostly benign; present with headaches, palpitations, episodic sweating
- **RCC and renal cysts** (found in 60% of patients):

- VHL disease is the most common cause of inherited RCC
- Many multiple and bilateral tumours. Usually asymptomatic
- **Pancreatic tumours**: usually asymptomatic
- Endolymphatic sac tumours (inner ear tumours): benign; however, the tumours can erode nearby bone:
  - Present with **hearing loss**, tinnitus, vertigo or facial weakness
- Pregnancy: hormonal and haemodynamic effects ↑haemangioblastoma growth → ↑symptom effects

INVESTIGATIONS

- Diagnosis is possible from the family history and genetic testing:
  - +ve family history + tumour
  - −ve family history + >2 CNS/retinal haemangioblastomas + visceral tumour
- Regular annual screening protocol:
  - Urinary metanephrines level (for phaeochromocytoma)
  - Abdominal and renal USS (show RCC and cysts)
  - Ophthalmic review (for retinal haemangioblastomas)
  - MRI brain spine (2–3 yearly; for CNS haemangioblastomas)
  - Auditory questionnaire: depending on the results, an audiogram +/- MRI should be considered (for endolymphatic sac tumours)
- Antenatal screening: if a VHL mutation is found in a family member

MANAGEMENT

- Annual screening: *see Investigations*
- Surgery: tumour resection (depending on type, size and location)
- Genetic counselling

COMPLICATIONS

These are dependent on the specific tumour presentation

PROGNOSIS

Previously life expectancy was ~50 y/o. The prognosis has improved with screening and current available treatments

WALLENBERG SYNDROME

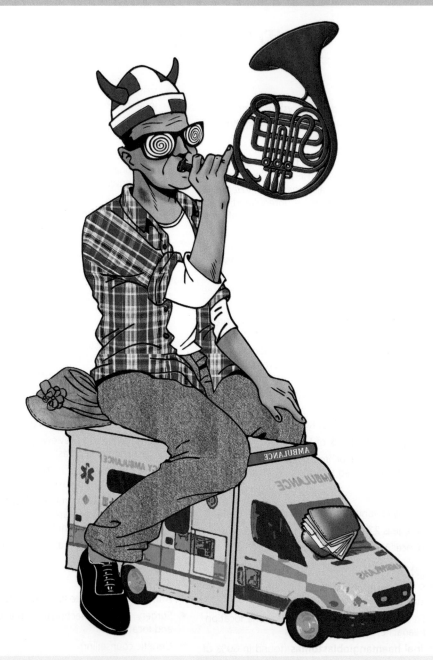

The ambulance has a stuffed wallet on its windscreen	**Wallenberg syndrome** Walle-t = Walle-nberg
He is sitting on a pink hat	**PICA (Posterior inferior cerebellar artery)** Pink-hat loosely sounds like PI-CA
He is wearing a hat with a Danish flag	**Cerebellar signs (DANISH)**
The man is blowing on a blue French horn	**Horner's syndrome**
He is sitting on top of an ambulance	**Nucleus ambiguus**
His sunglasses have a spiral pattern	**Vertigo**
He is wearing a check shirt	**Checkerboard pattern**
He has a large 'hickey' on the side of his neck	**Hickey = hiccups**

WALLENBERG SYNDROME

DEFINITION

PICA occlusion leading to lateral medulla (affecting multiple nuclei and inferior cerebellar peduncle) infarction. Hence, it is also known as lateral medullary syndrome

AETIOLOGY

- Anatomy: the **PICA** is the largest branch of the vertebral artery. PICA supplies the lateral medulla and inferior cerebellar peduncle on either side
- Pathophysiology: occlusion of either the vertebral artery or PICA will lead to infarction of multiple tracts and nuclei located in the lateral medulla and inferior cerebellar peduncle

EPIDEMIOLOGY

Rare; 20% of stroke cases occur in the vertebrobasilar circulation

PRESENTATION

- Clinical features correlate to the structures affected that are supplied by the **PICA**
- Ipsilateral features:
  - Inferior cerebellar peduncle → ipsilateral **cerebellar signs (DANISH)**: **D**ysdiadochokinesia, **A**taxia, **N**ystagmus, **I**ntention tremor, **S**lurred speech and **H**ypotonia
  - Descending sympathetic fibres → ipsilateral **Horner's syndrome**
  - **Nucleus ambiguus** (incorporate CN IX and X) → dysarthria, dysphagia:
    - Nucleus ambiguus involvement is specific to Wallenberg syndrome; the rest can be seen in lateral pontine syndrome (AICA occlusion)
  - Vestibular nucleus → nystagmus, **vertigo**, N&V
  - Spinal trigeminal nucleus → ipsilateral facial pain and temperature loss:
    - Receives pain and temperature sensation from the ipsilateral face
- Contralateral features:
  - Anterior spinothalamic tract → contralateral trunk and limb pain and temperature loss:
    - The tract decussates prior to moving up through the lateral medulla
- **Checkerboard pattern**: the loss of pain and temperature of the ipsilateral face and contralateral body helps facilitate the diagnosis of Wallenberg syndrome
- **Intermittent, violent hiccups**: the mechanism is poorly understood; it has been hypothesised that within the nucleus ambiguus lie vagal laryngeal motor neurons (that control the glottis) and premotor neurons (that control the inspiratory muscles). Hence, a lesion in this region → ↑activity of glottis and inspiratory muscles → ↑hiccups
- No muscle weakness as the medullary pyramids (through which the corticospinal tract travels) are not affected

INVESTIGATIONS

These are the same as for stroke

MANAGEMENT

These are the same as for stroke

COMPLICATIONS

These are the same as for stroke

PROGNOSIS

These are the same as for stroke

WERNICKE–KORSAKOFF SYNDROME

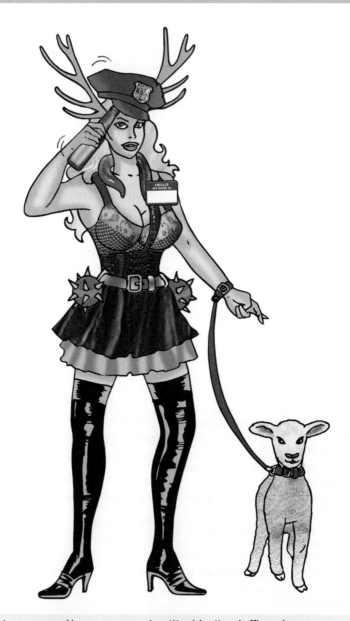

A female 'cop' is wearing a corset and has a worm around her neck	**Wernicke–Korsakoff's syndrome** Wernicke = worm; corset-cop = Korsakoff
She has land mines on her belt on her hips	**Thiamine**
She is wearing her bra outside of her uniform	**Mammillary bodies lesion**
She is walking her pet lamb	**Thalamic lesion**
She is scratching her head with an alcohol bottle	**Confusion, alcohol**
She has antlers on her head, and is unable to look laterally	**Ophthalmoplegia, nystagmus, lateral gaze palsy** Ny-'stag'-mus = have antlers
Her feet are spread widely apart	**Wide-based gait**
She has a name badge that is blank	**Amnesia** Unable to remember her name
She has the fingers on her left hand crossed	**Confabulation** Her fingers are crossed as she is being untruthful

WERNICKE–KORSAKOFF SYNDROME

DEFINITION

A spectrum of neurological disease due to thiamine deficiency, usually related to alcohol abuse and poor nutrition. It comprises acute Wernicke's encephalopathy and, if not treated, Korsakoff's syndrome, although both can occur separately

AETIOLOGY

- Pathophysiology: **thiamine** (vitamin B$_1$) is a co-factor for several key enzymes important in energy metabolism; deficiency due to alcohol excess/malnutrition leads to ATP depletion → the brain and heart are affected most (highly aerobic). This leads to petechial haemorrhages, astrocytosis and, if left untreated, neural death in the **mammillary bodies** and **thalamus** (areas of the brain with high thiamine usage and turnover, seen in Korsakoff's psychosis)
- Risk factors: classically it is associated with **alcoholism** (2° to ↓dietary intake, ↓gastric absorption, ↓hepatic storage and impaired utilisation). It is also seen in bariatric surgery, cancer, hyperemesis of pregnancy and starvation
- It can be exacerbated by high-dose glucose given prior to thiamine administration (see the mechanism described below):
  - Glucose → pyruvate (via the glycolysis pathway). Pyruvate → acetyl-CoA (by PDH; PDH uses thiamine as co-factor) → drives aerobic ATP formation
  - Giving glucose prior to thiamine in thiamine-deficient patient → ↑pyruvate (as PDH is unable to convert to acetyl-CoA) → ↓ATP formation. ↑Pyruvate in plasma is anaerobically converted into lactate → acidosis

EPIDEMIOLOGY

- Alcohol-related brain damage contributes between 10% and 25% of all cases of dementia
- Prevalence is higher in lower socio-economic areas, and in those 50–60 y/o

PRESENTATION

Wernicke's encephalopathy

- Classic triad (note not all do not necessarily occur in the same patient):
  - Encephalopathy; disorientation, inattentiveness, **confusion**, coma (90%)
  - **Ophthalmoplegia** (due to brainstem lesions): **nystagmus, lateral rectus palsy**, conjugate gaze palsies (96%):
    - Reflects involvement of the oculomotor, abducens and vestibular nuclei

- Ataxia (87%): **wide-based gait**; likely a combination of polyneuropathy, cerebellar and vestibular dysfunction

Korsakoff's psychosis

- Usually occurs in the 'resolution' phase of Wernicke's syndrome that was treated late or inadequately. Significant memory disorder with good preservation of other cognitive functions; cannot be reversed
- **Anterograde and retrograde amnesia**
- Horizontal nystagmus
- **Confabulation**: 'honest lying' – unconscious filling of gaps in memory by imagined or untrue experiences owing to retrograde amnesia. They have no conscious intention to deceive. Generally, patients are very confident about their recollections, despite contradictory evidence
- Apathy
- Lack of insight:
  - To diagnose Korsakoff's syndrome, the above features must persist beyond the usual duration of intoxication/withdrawal

INVESTIGATIONS

- A clinical diagnosis based on the presentation
- Bloods: plasma pyruvate, ↓RBC transketolase (↓ in thiamine deficiency, not usually necessary to diagnose)
- MRI brain: rules out structural lesions

MANAGEMENT

- A medical emergency
- Wernicke's encephalopathy: IV/IM high-dose **thiamine** (500 mg). Thiamine must be given before glucose to prevent neuronal death
- Korsakoff's syndrome: only 20% is reversible with thiamine. High-dose thiamine BD/TDS is given for 3–12 months
- MDT approach to include management of alcohol abuse

COMPLICATIONS

Other thiamine-deficiency conditions such as dry beriberi (neurological/muscular dysfunction) and wet beriberi (heart failure)

PROGNOSIS

- Death occurs in 20%
- 80% of Wernicke sufferers go on to develop Korsakoff's syndrome
- 25% of Korsakoff patients require long-term institutionalisation

INDEX

Printed and bound by CPI Group (UK) Ltd, Croydon, CR0 4YY

12/11/2024

01787613-0012